Natural Prozac

Also by Dr. Joel C. Robertson
and Tom Monte

Peak-Performance Living

Natural Prozac

Learning to Release Your Body's Own Anti-Depressants

Dr. Joel C. Robertson
with Tom Monte

HarperSanFrancisco
An Imprint of HarperCollins*Publishers*

HarperCollins Web Site: http://www.harpercollins.com
HarperCollins®, 📖®, and HarperSanFrancisco™
are trademarks of HarperCollins Publishers Inc.

FIRST EDITION

Library of Congress Cataloging-in-Publication Data
    Robertson, Joel C.
    Natural Prozac : learning to release your body's own anti-depressants / Joel C. Robertson
    with Tom Monte. — 1st ed.
    ISBN 0–06–251353–2 (cloth)
    ISBN 0–06–251354–0 (pbk.)
    1. Depression, Mental—Alternative treatment.   2. Depression, mental—Pathophysiology.
    I. Monte, Tom.   II. Title.
    RC537.R59   1997
    616.85'2706—dc20   96–33513

97 98 99 00 01 ❖RRDH 10 9 8 7 6 5 4 3 2 1

This book is dedicated to
Vickie, my wife,
to Nicole, Heidi, and Brooke,
my three lovely daughters,
and to the thousands suffering from depression

Contents

Acknowledgments

Through my work on the natural treatment of depression, I have become increasingly aware of how important and timely this topic is for today's society. My writer, Tom Monte, and I wanted to offer cutting-edge information that is based on research yet practical and easy to apply. This book is the result of our efforts. Although not all conservative clinicians will agree with everything we have written, we hope that they will see the value of moving from a "drug approach" to a "lifestyle approach" in treating depression.

A book of this magnitude requires the help of several people.

First I would like to thank my wife, Vickie, and my three daughters, Nicole, Heidi, and Brooke, for their energy and enthusiasm. As I worked with this sensitive and important subject, their enthusiasm for life gave me the energy I needed to keep pushing to completion.

I would also like to thank Tom Monte, an extraordinary person and writer, who continued to work on the manuscript in spite of issues relating to his mother's health, as well as other pressures. His drive to help others is greatly appreciated. This is his book as much as it is mine.

To the people of Harper Collins Publishers, my thanks. First to Tom Grady, executive editor, for his continued vision for my work.

Over the years that we have known each other, he has always encouraged me to bring my research to the public. To Caroline Pincus, an extraordinary editor, whose ability to make a book "read well" continues to amaze me. To the publicity and marketing department for their energy and creativity. To Nancy Palmer Jones and Rosana Francescato. And to all the others at Harper San Francisco for their talent and support.

Finally, I thank God for providing this opportunity to use the talents he has given me to help those who seek freedom from their depression and anxiety.

Thank you to all,
Joel C. Robertson

Foreword

found it somewhat overwhelming to write this book because of the complexity of the subject. Depression has a diversity of symptoms, multiplicity of causes, and wide range of effects on a person.

Although the brain is the center point of all depression, a person's genetic makeup, past history and environmental factors, lifestyle, food choices, and even thought processes affect their brain chemistry. Therefore we can have multiple causes with multiple factors influencing these causes.

In order to understand what causes the symptoms of depression, we must look at brain chemistry. By doing so, we can understand the causes of the symptoms and choose methods to alleviate such symptoms, in spite of the multiplicity of external or internal factors affecting the brain chemistry. In essence this means that even if a person's depression is inherited and they have been through major conflicts in their life, the one common factor is how both issues affect their brain chemistry. By focusing on brain chemistry, we can more accurately assess and deal with the other issues contributing to depression. One thing we know for sure is that feelings of hopelessness and negativity must be resolved to overcome depression. Since hopelessness and negativity are symptoms of altered brain chemistry, we must address brain chemistry first in order for other methods to be helpful.

It was also difficult to write about our society's attitudes toward using medication. I often hear colleagues or clients speak of their desire for anti-depressants. I also am well aware of the tremendous effect of anti-depressants on behavior, anxiety, and depression. However, I urge you to consider this one simple point: *Medications don't change behavior, the effect medication has on brain chemistry changes behavior.* Essentially, this means that changing brain chemistry changes behavior. The assumption that medication is necessary to change brain chemistry is erroneous. It may be the quickest and easiest method, but it is not the only way to alter brain chemistry. It certainly is not the safest.

We have known for many years that various foods, activities, behaviors, and even thoughts alter brain chemistry. Anyone who has eaten a large meal in the afternoon has felt the effect of altered brain chemicals a couple of hours later. The sluggishness or tiredness is caused by altered brain chemistry. The "runner's high" and decrease in feelings of stress associated with exercise has been well documented. Again, it is the effect of exercise on brain chemicals that has altered the feelings. Conflict, procrastination, overeating, and other behaviors can cause us to be anxious, stressed, or depressed, all symptoms of altered brain chemistry. Even thoughts and emotions, such as fear, frustration, insecurity, or anger, alter our brain chemistry. These changes in brain chemistry often create negative behaviors. For example, we are all aware of how anger can affect our perception (a result of altered brain chemicals) and our behaviors. We know that behaviors, diet, activities, and thoughts can change our brain chemistry negatively or positively. The choice to make their effects positive is dependent on your knowledge of the brain chemicals you need to change.

Therefore, if we know that these factors alter brain chemicals and that depression is the result of altered brain chemicals, it makes sense to tailor activity, diet, behaviors, and thoughts to make specific brain chemistry changes. The key is knowing which *specific* chemicals need to be enhanced or reduced and which behaviors will do that. If you can understand which chemicals are primarily responsible for your feelings of depression, compulsions, or even anxiety, then you can tailor your recovery program. That is the purpose of this book.

I would be remiss if I did not recognize that some individuals will require medication to get over their hopelessness and begin to make changes. That does not mean that they need medication permanently. It may be a "jump start" to their recovery. If you require medication, you can begin to follow the program described in this book and work with your physician to begin to taper or perhaps even eliminate the use of medication altogether.

In this book I have attempted to gather what is known about the brain, simplify the complexity of the brain into a usable format, and provide clear-cut choices for tailoring a recovery program. I believe the research done in the conservative medical community backs up the information in this book. I am aware that I have one simple difference with their conclusions: medication doesn't cure depression—it alters brain chemistry, which cures depression. Medication is only one of the methods to alter brain chemistry. For me, and I hope for you, the best way to change brain chemistry is the healthiest and longest-acting method, not the quickest and possibly the most dangerous.

Please understand one more very important point before you begin on a journey of self-prescribed recovery. If you are on medication or are feeling hopeless, work with a physician on tapering your medication or to evaluate your need for medication to get you "on your feet." Depression can be dangerous and rob you of joy needlessly. Although the methods described in this book will help most people improve, some will need medication and counseling to recover fully. I urge you to make that choice sooner rather than later. It is much easier to recover in the earlier stages of depression than in the later stages.

May God bless you in your endeavor to achieve a healthy and fulfilling life.

Dr. Joel Robertson

Natural Prozac

Introduction

The human brain is an organ of limitless complexity and wonder, a universe found within the confines of blood, nerves, and bone. More than any other organ, the brain is associated with all those invisible aspects of our humanness that determine the quality of our lives, including our psychological condition and, specifically, our moods. The mediators of mood, the very substances that create it, are an array of brain chemicals called *neurotransmitters*. Certain neurotransmitters can become imbalanced and cause a variety of psychological conditions, including depression. Yet not only can these neurotransmitters be restored to harmony but they can also provide each of us with a more balanced perspective on life, with a deeper sense of contentment, and with more happiness and joy. In this book, I will show you how to restore the balance of these brain chemicals in order to alleviate and even overcome depression.

A great deal has been written and said about depression, and much of it is pretty disheartening to anyone who suffers from this condition. Scientists, psychologists, and psychiatrists are nearly as frustrated by depression as are its sufferers.

Since the 1950s we have used medication to alter brain chemistry, which in turn changes behaviors and feeling. Thorazine, a medication from the '50s, affected dopamine levels, which helped to clear up the symptoms of schizophrenia. However, the side effects of lethargy, unclear thinking, and unresponsiveness to emotions were less than optimal. In the '60s and '70s, drugs such as Valium and anti-depressants, such as Elavil and Triavil, became available. Again, their side effects of drowsiness and unclear thinking encouraged researchers to continue to search for new anti-depressants. The 1990s have brought us into an era of newer anti-depressants, such as Prozac, which are more selective in targeting a specific neurotransmitter. For example, most of the newer anti-depressants are more selective than older ones in affecting serotonin levels. However, serotonin affects not only moods but also many other things, such as vision, functioning of the gastrointestinal tract, perception, and memory. So even these newer drugs have side effects, such as drowsiness, which are really the effects of raising serotonin levels artificially. Some of these effects may seem minor, but when something like our perception is changed, that can affect our relationships, our understanding of ourselves, and even our spiritual life. To avoid these side effects, we need to alter our brain chemistry naturally when at all possible. I believe this should be the goal of even those who benefit from anti-depressants.

Drug treatments do relieve the symptoms of depression in about a third of all cases, but many people fail to respond to pharmaceuticals, and others experience disturbing side effects. Equally troubling is the fact that drug treatments usually don't address the source of the depression, which means that if people go off their medication, the depression often comes back. Thus, many depressed people are expected to stay on anti-depressants for the rest of their lives.

Some of these people are also frustrated by psychotherapy, in part because it takes so long and sometimes because they have not found a therapist who truly understands depression and has an effective approach to treating it. Interestingly, when psychotherapy succeeds, it is because the patient has looked at his or her patterns of behavior and made behavioral changes. What's really going on, as I will demonstrate, is that the right behavioral changes actually alter brain chemistry—they can even do it pretty rapidly—and thus they reduce or eliminate the symptoms of depression. Without a knowledge of brain chemistry, many therapists don't understand the kinds of behavioral modifications that are necessary to make these changes in the brain and then sustain them. For instance, this book maintains that there are two major types of depression, which I refer to as Satiation depression and Arousal depression. These two types of depression will be defined in detail as we go along, but the point here is that one set of behaviors helps to overcome the Satiation type, while another works for the Arousal type—*and the tools for healing each type of depression are not interchangeable.* Unless we have a clear understanding of a depressed person's brain chemistry, we may recommend behaviors that will seem to be therapeutic but that are in fact only reinforcing the underlying brain-chemistry imbalance, which is causing the depression in the first place. In this book I will show you how to pinpoint which type of depression you, or someone you love, may be suffering from, and I will suggest which tools to use to treat it.

How many depressed people have been told to "just cheer up"? But if depressed people could "just cheer up," they would have done it a long time ago. People who are not depressed often do not understand how difficult it is for a depressed person to start feeling or thinking differently. Depressed people cannot simply "cheer up," because they suffer from a chemical imbalance in their central nervous system that is the source of their depression. Fortunately, balance can be restored, and that is the aim of this book. Just as a person's experiences and behavior can create the kinds of chemical imbalances that give rise to depression, so their experiences and behaviors can also restore chemical balance. And only by restoring chemical balance can we truly hope to *cure* depression.

The underlying theory in this book is based on just these two ideas: (1) the chemicals in our brain help to create our feelings, moods, thoughts, and behavior; and (2) our brain chemistry is altered by food, exercise, thoughts, emotions, and actions. This is what I call the *brain-chemistry model.* Unbeknownst to most of us, we are constantly changing our brain chemistry every day. Unfortunately, because we do not realize how powerful the effect of our behavior is on brain chemistry, we tend to continue behaviors that sustain depression. Small changes in behavior can cause significant changes in brain chemistry and mood. By altering your behavior, you can dramatically improve your psychological and emotional health. In this book, I will show how all of us alter our brain chemistry to create our internal psychological state. And I will demonstrate how common behaviors can either maintain a brain-chemical imbalance and thus sustain depression—or be used to balance our brain chemicals in order to overcome depression.

As a clinician and an expert in pharmacology and brain chemistry, I have worked with more than ten thousand people with a wide range of psychological and neurochemical conditions. This work has helped me to understand the effects of individual behaviors and foods on brain chemistry, and as a result, I have been able to group activities and foods into well-designed programs that boost specific brain chemicals. These programs are safe, natural, and nontoxic. In fact, they are made up of ordinary behaviors and common foods. I have been developing and using these programs for the last twenty years and have found them to be remarkably effective.

In fact, the brain-chemistry model is amazingly egalitarian: it works for the vast majority of people. It also reveals why drug therapy succeeds in some cases and doesn't in others. It shows us why certain forms of psychotherapy can be very effective in helping to treat depression. And it demonstrates how our own attitudes, misperceptions, dietary practices, and behavioral patterns can create depression and—most important—how food, exercise, and other behaviors can help us overcome it.

Balance as the Key to Health and Healing

The key to health—from both a biochemical and a psychological perspective—is balance. Without balance, we have extremes in behavior and brain chemistry, and these extremes create the basis for negative feelings and behaviors of one kind or another.

My work has led me to distinguish between two types of personalities, which I call the Satiation personality and the Arousal personality. Satiation types prefer quiet and calm to a lot of excitement, while Arousal types tend to be excitable, high-energy people. When we become too much of one type to the exclusion of the other, we establish a brain-chemistry imbalance that forms the basis for depression. If you are by nature a Satiation type, for example, you may risk becoming too passive, accepting, and security conscious; these attitudes may put you in danger of becoming depressed and of not being able to find a way out of that depression. On the other hand, if you are an Arousal type, you may risk becoming too goal-oriented, and you may experience excess stress, anxiety, and fear; this pattern, too, can lead to depression. Arousal types will often be more aware of their anxiety than of their depression; indeed, this is usually one of the reasons they choose a high-anxiety lifestyle: to avoid feeling their depression.

Fortunately, the behavioral changes that I recommend for each of these personality types are small and effective in the short term. People who adopt my program can find relief from their symptoms within a relatively short period of time.

But all of this does mean that a depressed person's participation is essential to overcoming his or her condition. And this can be awfully tough, I know. Yet behavior change must occur in order for you to feel better. My central premise in this book is that depression is the result of an *imbalance* in our approach to life—an imbalance that gives rise to chemical changes in the brain and central nervous system—and these chemical changes create and support depression. Healing depression, then, is a matter of *restoring balance* to the brain chemistry through the use of food, exercise, thoughts, and behavioral change.

But the brain-chemistry model is not just a means of reducing us all to a finite set of chemicals and nerve cells. I see the brain as a tool of the *mind*—that infinite expanse within us often referred to as the psyche. The word *psyche* in Greek means breath, life, spirit. Thus, people have always known intuitively that the mind is the gateway to the spirit. Yes, the mind provides us with the intellectual capabilities essential for survival. But the riches of the psyche lie in its deeper realms, where we find the gifts of contentment, compassion, and the ability to give life meaning and purpose. This book approaches the subject of healing depression through the body, mind, and spirit. Such an understanding, I feel, is essential. At the same time, I hope that this book will inspire in you the same awe that I feel for this remarkable organ, the brain—the physical matrix where body, mind, and spirit become one.

Part 1 Understanding
the Roots of
Depression

Chapter 1

The Challenges of Treating Depression

Understanding the Brain and Depression

In the blink of an eye, your brain interprets every experience you have and responds physically, intellectually, and emotionally, sending you a message that is at once infinitely complex and as simple as a single thought: "I feel good" or "happy" or "sad" or "safe" or "afraid" or "depressed." All your memories, abilities, talents, weaknesses, and potential as a human being lie within your brain. Everything you have ever experienced and learned —indeed, your very identity—is recorded in the tissues of a three-pound sphere that is really neither very pretty nor very big.

When you think about all the jobs your brain performs—well, your brain can get tired just thinking about them. A short list doesn't come close to being representative, though it does provide a basis for our awe. The brain is the regulating center of the body, interpreting billions of bits of information received from the body and your environment and then offering a staggering array of biological, intellectual, and emotional reactions too numerous and complex to name. The brain is the seat of consciousness, that state of awareness that tells us who we are, where we are, and what is happening around us. The brain is the receiver and interpreter of the senses. Everything we see, hear, touch, taste, and smell—no matter whether these stimuli come from within the body or outside it—is recorded and understood by the brain. The brain controls all the involuntary actions that are responsible for maintaining life within the body, such as your heartbeat, nerve function, hormonal activity, immune function, assimilation of oxygen and nutrition, and elimination of waste. Every conscious and unconscious act that you perform is initiated by your brain. The brain is the seat of all intellectual activity. It also mediates all your emotional experiences and instinctive drives, such as hunger, rest, sleep, touch, sex, and companionship. And the brain is responsible for regulating your moods, including joy, hope, and depression.

The *American Medical Association Encyclopedia of Medicine* defines depression as "feelings of sadness, hopelessness, pessimism, and a general loss of interest in life, combined with a sense of reduced emotional well-being." Other authorities state that depression is associated with sleep disturbances, with loss of concentration, energy, appetite, and activity, and with withdrawal from social behavior. People who are depressed typically feel hopeless and suffer from low self-esteem. Many lose weight; others gain weight. Some describe depression as a feeling of "emptiness" or "being numb." Some say that they have no feelings at all. Depression can suppress the immune system and result in generalized fatigue and exhaustion. Those who suffer from severe depression—a condition known as "major depression"—can experience hallucinations, delusions, and recurrent deep-seated guilt.

It is easy to see that depression has a widespread effect on brain function. In fact, when we consider all the physical and psychological symptoms associated with depression and then review all the things that the brain does, we get a clear picture of how pervasive depression's effects can be on the brain and thus on your entire life. Depression, then, has its roots in this remarkable organ.

Obviously, the challenge in treating depression is understanding this complex brain and trying to put it in balance. That is precisely why it should be done naturally. Every time we alter one effect artificially, we create change in another area. The challenge then becomes changing the negative brain issues specifically for me, not a depressed society or group of people, but me—my specific brain and my specific issues. This is a challenge, but it is not insurmountable.

The connection between the dark cloud of depression and the physical brain lies in a set of neurotransmitters. These neurotransmitters are actually messenger chemicals that create feelings, stimulate thoughts, and trigger memories, just to name a few of the things they do. When you have an optimal amount of any single neurotransmitter in your brain, then you will experience the positive feelings associated with that neurotransmitter. A deficiency or excess of any single neurotransmitter usually results in the negative experiences associated with that brain chemical.

In this book, I'm going to discuss five of these neurotransmitters: serotonin, dopamine, norepinephrine, acetylcholine, and gamma-aminobutyric acid (or GABA). Of these five, three are of particular importance in depression: serotonin, norepinephrine, and dopamine.

Your brain chemistry changes depending on your thoughts, expectations, and activities, the foods you eat, and the kinds of exercises you perform. In fact, every single physical act, thought, emotion, and image you call to mind triggers a corresponding change in your brain chemistry.

Yet despite the fact that brain chemistry can undergo such significant changes, all of us—no matter what our mood is at any given moment—tend to maintain an internal chemical balance within pretty specific limits. We do this by maintaining a certain consistency in the ways we think, eat, and behave each day. I call this consistent pattern your *brain-chemistry baseline*, or simply your *baseline*. In fact, you maintain your sense of identity by maintaining your baseline.

Depression, as I've said, is the result of an imbalance in the chemical combination in your brain. This imbalance can become your baseline; in other words, some people's identities can become associated with depression. These people maintain their long-standing depression by sustaining the ways in which they think, eat, behave, and interact with others. Throughout this book, I will be talking about personality types that, taken to the extreme, support depression. You will have to look inside yourself to see whether these descriptions fit you and to determine which elements in your personality and behavior might be keeping you from achieving your optimal level of well-being.

Obviously, many depressed people do not have to look very hard to find the cause of their depression. The loss of a job or spouse or some other traumatic event can trigger a life crisis that may include depression. Such events can and do actually change our brain chemistry. Unless we fully grieve our losses, allowing ourselves to feel the pain until we are able to let it go, we can get stuck in such feelings and have trouble moving on. In such cases, the brain chemistry may establish a new pattern—a new baseline—that actually supports chronic or long-standing depression.

But loss is only one cause of depression. Some people have genetic imbalances that predispose them to depression. Others come from families in which there was abuse or some other behavioral pattern that has promoted the onset of depression later in life. Still others suffer from depression but cannot pinpoint its origins. I will discuss all of these types of depression later in this book.

For now, you should understand that no matter what the cause of your melancholy or despair, such feelings are rooted in a neurochemical imbalance in your brain. *You have the power to restore harmony and balance to these neurotransmitters and in the process alleviate and overcome your depressed feelings.*

Through a variety of natural, health-promoting activities and choices, I will provide you with new ways of understanding yourself and your behavior and ways of dealing with situations and emotions that can help you avoid depression. These tools all change your brain chemistry, and in many cases, they do it rapidly. By changing your brain chemistry, you can create a more harmonious and uplifting frame of mind.

Boosting Brain Chemistry: Drugs Versus Behavioral Change

Currently, the drugs used to treat depression are designed to affect three chemical neurotransmitters. The first of these is *serotonin*, a neurotransmitter that boosts feelings of optimism, well-being, self-esteem, relaxation, and security. Serotonin improves our ability to concentrate on a particular problem; it also enhances sleep. When serotonin is optimal, people tend to be relaxed. They experience little or no anxiety or fear. When serotonin levels are low, depression is common; the person may also suffer from poor sleep and an inability to concentrate. Scientists at the University of California at Los Angeles and other research centers have shown that people who are chronically low in serotonin are often chronically depressed; some are prone to violence against both others and themselves. Very few people have naturally high levels of serotonin. Rather, most people have moderate to normal levels of serotonin, and this helps them avoid depression. The most commonly prescribed pharmaceuticals designed to treat depression—such as Prozac, Zoloft, and Paxil—raise serotonin levels in the brain in order to improve a person's mood and enhance feelings of well-being.

The other two neurotransmitters affected by drugs are *dopamine* and its derivative, *norepinephrine*. They are often considered a single chemical, since one is a derivative of the other, and referred to simply as norepinephrine. These two neurotransmitters increase feelings of alertness, assertiveness, aggression, and wakefulness. They heighten energy, speed up thoughts, and improve muscle coordination. Low brain levels of dopamine and norepinephrine can cause depression. Conversely, higher than normal levels create anxiety and, in some people, cause aggression; excessively high levels of these two neuro-transmitters can give rise to violent behavior, schizophrenia, paranoia, and other forms of psychosis. When serotonin is low and dopamine and norepinephrine are high, a person can experience both depression and anxiety, a very common condition.

A group of pharmaceutical drugs called *tricyclic anti-depressants* overcome depression by boosting norepinephrine, dopamine, and sero-tonin, thereby raising energy levels and restoring a stronger sense of self and sense of purpose. Among the most commonly prescribed are Elavil, Triavil, Amoxapine, and Doxepin. A newer drug, called Well-butin, also falls into this category but has lesser effects on serotonin.

As these descriptions suggest, it is easy to divide these three neu-rotransmitters into two groups. I refer to the first one, serotonin, as a "well-being" brain chemical because it creates feelings of relaxation and a certain degree of passivity, in addition to improving concentra-tion. The second group consists of dopamine and norepinephrine, which create alertness and aggression. They give rise to action and ex-citement, so I refer to these two as "energizer" brain chemicals.

This book offers a natural, nondrug approach to healing depression. However, there are occasions when drug therapy is essential, at least for a while. During this period, other therapies can be used in con-junction with the pharmaceuticals to help alleviate depression. The following questionnaire will help you understand your conditions and emotions better; it will also help you determine whether you should be seeking professional help and perhaps taking medication for your condition.

➤ Depressive Index:
A Guide to Help You Determine Your Emotional Condition and Course of Treatment

Answer "mostly yes" or "mostly no" to the following questions.

1. Do you feel depressed most of the day?
2. Do you feel depressed almost every day?
3. Do you get little or no pleasure from any activities you do?
4. Have you lost weight (more than 5 percent of body weight) within a thirty-day period?
5. Have you gained weight (more than 5 percent of body weight) within a thirty-day period (unless related to pregnancy)?
6. Do you have difficulty getting to sleep nearly every day?
7. Do you have feel you sleep too much nearly every day?
8. Do you have a loss of energy nearly every day?
9. Do you have feelings of worthlessness or excessive guilt nearly every day?
10. Do you have difficulty thinking or concentrating nearly every day, or has your ability to think and concentrate diminished recently?
11. Do you have recurrent thoughts of death or suicide?

Evaluating Your Answers

Count up the number of "yes" answers you gave to these questions.

If you had more than five "yes" answers, you should seek professional help. You may be suffering a major depression. This book may offer assistance as you work with your physician or counselor, but you may also need medication to help you during the initial phases of recovery.

If you gave three to five "yes" answers, you may or may not require professional help. If you have any recurrent thoughts of suicide or your depression worsens, you should seek professional help.

One or two "yes" answers indicate a mild depression (professional help may or may not be required). If you have any recurrent thoughts of suicide or your depression worsens, you should seek professional help. But this book is a great starting point for you.

If you answer "yes" to any of the following questions, please seek professional help.

- Do you have distinct periods of abnormally and persistently elevated moods that cause you to experience grandiosity (the feeling of being more powerful than you are), decreased need for sleep, racing thoughts, agitation, or participation in plea-surable activities that are self-destructive?
- Does your mood prevent you from going to work or function-ing at your occupation?
- Have you experienced delusions or hallucinations during your mood changes?
- Do you have a preexisting medical disorder that has precipi-tated your depression?

If the results indicate that you are severely depressed or if you have answered "yes" to any of the additional questions, this book by it-self is not for you. I urge you to talk to a physician or a psychiatrist. You may then use the principles in this book while also following your doctor's advice on medication or therapy.

The Limitations of Drugs in Treating Depression

No one should approach the subject of depression without a healthy respect both for the condition itself and for those who struggle with it. I will not trivialize how difficult depression is to deal with and overcome. Nor do I offer my programs blithely, as if they provided a simple how-to formula for dealing with everyone's condition. There are no easy answers for depression. The programs I suggest require effort and change. By following these recommendations, you, or someone you care about who may be suffering from depression, can alter the current combination of neurotransmitters that are supporting your condition. In the process, you can boost those brain chemicals that create feelings of well-being, high self-esteem, relaxation, and confidence.

Right now many researchers are working feverishly to figure out new and better approaches to depression. My own work would not be possible without the research that has been done on brain chemistry. As our understanding of how the brain works has increased, our dependence on drug therapy has grown even stronger because we know that altering brain chemistry improves depression. Today, physicians emphasize anti-depressive drugs as the primary treatment for depression. Yet virtually everyone in the fields of psychology, psychiatry, and pharmacology will tell you that none of these drugs is a cure for depression, and many can have harmful side effects. In fact, more and more scientists are questioning our reliance on pharmaceuticals as the primary treatment for depression. As Dr. Roger Greenburg, a psychologist in the Department of Psychiatry at the State University of New York Health Center in Syracuse, told the *New York Times:* "The answer to all psychiatric problems does not lie in drugs. The magnitude of their effect is far less than the public has been led to believe."

Despite the celebration in the popular press about the new wave of anti-depressant wonder drugs—the most widely touted being Prozac—studies have shown that these drugs do not have the salutary effects that the press reports. Prozac has only a "modest" effect on depression, according to a large-scale analysis of its effects (called a meta-analysis) published in the *Journal of Nervous and Mental Disease* (October 1994). The track records of other pharmaceuticals are not much better. At the same time, all anti-depressants have side effects, and for some people these side effects can be severe. It has been shown that the drugs that have the biggest impact on a patient's psychological state also have the most severe side effects. In the case of Prozac, those side effects span a wide spectrum of symptoms, ranging from nervous system disorders, anxiety, drowsiness, and loss of strength and energy to gastrointestinal disorders, nausea, diarrhea, and dizziness. In men, the drug can cause impotence. In some patients, Prozac increases obsessive thinking and thoughts of suicide.

As I have said, there are times when drugs are essential in the treatment process. In many instances, drugs not only enhance the patient's quality of life but actually save lives by preventing suicide and violent behavior. But our drug-dependent society must begin to recognize the limits of these pharmaceuticals and, whenever possible, stress nondrug treatments for psychological problems, including depression. We must achieve a more balanced approach that includes drug therapy when it is necessary but that relies just as heavily on behavioral change whenever possible. And as I have said, behavioral change is essential if we are to change the underlying brain chemistry that supports depression.

For Those Receiving Professional Help

In this book, I offer dietary and behavioral methods that can reduce depression and, for many, eliminate the condition entirely. These methods are not for everyone. Some people do not want to change their behavior. Others may want to read this book, consider their options, and talk to their physicians or therapists before deciding what's right for them. For those who want to use the programs I offer, you should understand that it doesn't matter whether or not you are on medication. You can still follow the program that is appropriate for you, as long as you do it under the supervision of your doctor. (Chapters Three, Four, and Five will help you decide which of the programs you need.) Ask your doctor to monitor your progress; you may be able to decrease your medication gradually and eventually stop it altogether as a result of the improvements you experience from the program. No matter whether you are seeing a psychiatrist or psychologist, whether you are taking psychoactive drugs or not, the programs described in this book can help you because they do precisely what the drugs are trying to do: increase or moderate certain chemicals in your brain.

Using Behaviors to Change Brain Chemistry

During the past twenty years, science has learned that neurotransmitters can be raised or lowered, often dramatically, by a wide variety of everyday behaviors. One of the most powerful—and fastest—ways to change our neurotransmitters is to change our food choices. Science has demonstrated that brain chemistry can be changed significantly by a single meal. This is a conclusion reached by most researchers in this field.

"It is becoming increasingly clear that brain chemistry and function can be influenced by a single meal," wrote Massachusetts Institute of Technology scientist John D. Fernstrom, Ph.D. "That is, in well-nourished individuals consuming normal amounts of food, short-term changes in food composition can rapidly affect brain function." Without knowing it, many depressed people are actually maintaining their depressions by continuing to eat certain foods and by maintaining certain behaviors.

Thus, drugs are not the only way to change brain chemistry dramatically. All three of the major neurotransmitters are altered by our daily behavior. If you go to a carnival or a circus, the sudden rush of activity that confronts your senses and nervous system will cause dopamine and norepinephrine levels in your brain to soar within minutes. The result is that you feel alert and excited. Put some of your favorite rock and roll on your stereo and try to sit still. Norepinephrine and dopamine are flooding your brain, causing your muscles to want to move, your respiration to increase, and your heart rate to accelerate. You may tell your partner that the music's beat is forcing you to dance, but actually the rhythms of norepinephrine are just as big a part of your inspiration. The same is true if you exercise. Play tennis or basketball or racquetball for an hour and you will boost your dopamine and norepinephrine levels significantly. During the workout, you will be alert, aggressive, and excited. After it, you'll be more relaxed, alert, and focused, thanks in part to the fact that you have used up dopamine and norepinephrine and your serotonin levels are now on the rise. Thus, knowing that behaviors affect our brain chemistry, we can use them to help us enhance our moods.

You can also boost dopamine and norepinephrine by eating foods rich in protein. The body converts protein into an amino acid called *tyrosine*, which is further converted into dopamine and norepinephrine in your brain. A single high-protein meal will raise your levels of norepinephrine and dopamine within minutes. In the process, you will be increasing your assertiveness, your alertness, and the speed of your thoughts.

Similarly, you can use behavior to boost serotonin levels. Go to a restaurant with a comfortable atmosphere or listen to some Chopin, soft jazz, or folk music, and you will quickly raise the levels of serotonin in your brain. Serotonin can also be increased by eating foods that are rich in carbohydrates. Carbohydrates enhance the absorption of an amino acid called *tryptophan*, which is converted into serotonin in the brain. Within minutes of eating a carbohydrate-rich food, such as a whole grain, whole-grain flour product, or even sugar, we experience significantly increased levels of serotonin. This is why so many of us are habitual sugar eaters. But as I will show later on, sugar is not the best way to maintain consistent serotonin levels. Our cells burn sugar rapidly; once the sugar levels drop, the serotonin levels also fall, which means that habitual sugar consumption can actually contribute to depression. The best way to consume carbohydrates is to eat whole grains, such as brown rice, oats, barley, corn, millet, quinoa, and amaranth or whole-wheat bread or noodles. These grains provide long chains of carbohydrates that are broken down in the intestinal tract and thus are secreted into your bloodstream over a long period of time. This constant flow of carbohydrates into your bloodstream creates a corresponding flow of serotonin into your nervous system and brain. The results are consistent feelings of well-being and greater concentration, confidence, and relaxation.

Combining Drug Treatment with Behavioral Change

It is in our power to change the levels of these chemicals in our brain at any time of the day. In fact, we do it all the time. Unfortunately, we typically fall into the patterns of behavior that reinforce the current brain-chemical configuration, and this in turn reinforces our mood and psychological state. In other words, because we resist change, we remain stuck with the same brain chemical imbalance and the same emotional condition.

Here's a crucial fact that you must understand in order to overcome depression: *Drugs designed to treat depression change the levels of these neurotransmitters in your brain without requiring you to change your behavior.* In other words, drugs make modest to dramatic changes in the feelings you experience without requiring you to change your way of life. Yet for a great many people who are depressed, it is their way of life that supports and nurtures the depression.

Studies have shown that when drugs are combined with psychotherapy, the effects are usually greater and have more lasting positive results than if drugs are used alone. A study published in the October 1989 issue of the *American Journal of Psychiatry* demonstrated that people who were severely depressed and were treated with both drugs and psychotherapy were psychologically healthier a year later than those who were treated with drugs alone. Even more significant is a study done by the National Institute of Mental Health that compared drug treatment with psychotherapy for people who were depressed. The study showed that the drug (imipramine) alone worked faster than the psychotherapy. However, after sixteen weeks researchers found that there was no difference in effect between the drugs and the psychotherapy. Other studies have shown that psychotherapy is better at preventing a relapse of depression than drugs are.

Now we must ask, Why were both treatments comparable after about four months? And why is it that psychotherapy takes longer but is more effective in the long run? Here are the answers:

Drugs change brain chemistry immediately, but because they do not require behavioral change, your daily actions continue to support your current out-of-balance brain chemistry, and this maintains your depression. This may be why many people continue to experience some mild form of depression, melancholy, or despair even when they are taking anti-depressants. In any case, as long as you haven't changed your behavior, you will continue to need those drugs because the underlying condition has not been altered. The drugs are merely masking the underlying condition; they are not curing it. The moment you stop the drugs, you will probably experience a relapse into depression.

Psychotherapy takes longer to create an improvement because it actually changes your behavior and outlook on life, and this in turn causes your brain chemistry to change. By changing the brain chemistry, you are healing the underlying conditions that are causing your depression. When you maintain your new, healthy behaviors consistently, you are actually changing what I call your *baseline* brain chemistry, which means you are positively altering the balance of your neurotransmitters. In short, you are curing your depression. This is why psychotherapy has been shown to be more effective at preventing a relapse of depression: because the new underlying brain chemistry is supporting emotional equilibrium. Your behavior has changed your brain chemistry for the good!

The programs I offer work much faster than many forms of psychotherapy alone, in part because they engage you in behaviors that change your brain chemistry immediately. This is not a criticism of psychotherapy. I think that therapy, like drug treatment, is essential for many people, especially because it gets people to confront behaviors that are causing their problems and helps them to change those behaviors. Good psychotherapy stimulates many of the behavioral changes that I also recommend to overcome depression. But in order to create rapid changes in brain chemistry and mood, you must focus on modifying certain behaviors, such as dietary choices and exercise. Often, such modifications are not encouraged by psychotherapists, which is why changes in mood occur more slowly with psychotherapy alone. For those in therapy, my programs will help you to make more rapid progress in your growth—and especially in your journey out of depression.

Identifying Which Behaviors to Change

No matter what your current health status is, your personality is probably dominated by one of the following brain-chemical configurations:

- Low levels of serotonin
- Low levels of dopamine and norepinephrine
- Low levels of both
- Low levels of serotonin and high levels of norepinephrine and dopamine

The predominance of one or another of these chemical combinations will give rise to very different personality characteristics. By looking at the kinds of behaviors that dominate your life, you can get a pretty accurate picture of which neurotransmitters are out of balance. This book provides a series of questionnaires to help you determine which of your neurotransmitters may be imbalanced. In Chapters Three, Four, and Five, I describe the personality types and their corresponding types of depression that are the result of certain neurotransmitter imbalances. I will ask you to decide which of these best describes your current condition. Once you know the type of personality you are, you will be able to decide which program suits you best. If you aren't depressed, these programs can help you to optimize your moods, decrease mood swings, and give you a greater sense of peace.

These programs can protect a person from becoming depressed. Since the programs are natural and nontoxic, you will benefit even if you choose the wrong one. All the programs boost serotonin, in addition to altering other brain chemicals, and as you will learn, all of us benefit by boosting serotonin.

Before we describe the personality types and their corresponding programs, however, we need to understand the brain and the neurotransmitters that trigger our moods and thinking a little better.

Chapter 2

The Biochemical
Roots of Depression

Valerie came from a seemingly perfect family. Her father was a medical doctor, her mother a loving and attentive homemaker. The family lived in the suburbs in an expensive home. Valerie got good grades in high school, went to college, and became homecoming queen and won the congeniality award. After college, she married an ambitious professional and started her own career as a real estate agent. To the casual observer, Valerie came from the ideal background and then achieved her own ideal lifestyle.

A few years after she was married, however, she was deeply depressed, quit her career, and believed her life would end tragically. She became addicted to alcohol and cigarettes and was eating compulsively. The young woman who had accomplished so much in high school, college, and her professional life had collapsed. What had happened?

Obviously, perfect images do not mean perfect lives, and on closer examination Valerie's childhood was anything but perfect. Her father's medical practice was so demanding that he rarely had any time to spend with his wife or his daughter, and this hurt both women. Valerie began to realize that it was not just her father's job that kept him away. She was sure that he simply didn't want to be home with his wife and daughter. Perhaps it was her mother's fault that he stayed away, or maybe it was Valerie herself. But it was clear that John didn't want to be a father and husband. His unwillingness to communicate exactly why he fled made it all the worse because Valerie ended up blaming herself for her father's absence. She loved her father deeply and wanted him to be around, so she felt abandoned and betrayed by him.

So did Valerie's mother. The two women provided each other with some emotional support, but nothing was going to replace John's presence. Moreover, Nancy, Valerie's mother, was angry at her husband for abandoning them. She and John raged at each other at times, but no matter what Nancy did, John remained remote and inaccessible to both Nancy and Valerie. Nancy's intense emotions added to the strain Valerie felt during her childhood and adolescence.

Through most of Valerie's young adulthood, her mother was depressed. Nancy managed to keep her addictions well hidden, at least to the outside world, but at home she was miserable most of the time. Valerie felt her mother's pain vicariously, but there was nothing she could do except suffer it with her. As a means of coping, Valerie tried to become the image of perfection at school; she was pretty, got good grades, and was popular. She entered college and carried off the same performance. But shortly after she got married, she fell into her mother's pattern: soon she was depressed and reluctant to leave her house. She started engaging in self-destructive behavior.

When I asked Valerie about her marriage, she described a loving, supportive husband. Yet she believed that he would become the same kind of man that her father was—obsessed with his career and bored by his family. In the end, she firmly believed that her life would be tragic, as her mother's had been. There was nothing she could do to change her fate, she believed. Such an attitude enveloped her like a toxic cloud and caused her to retreat ever more deeply from the outside world.

On a biochemical level, Valerie's beliefs had an effect on her brain chemistry, specifically lowering serotonin and norepinephrine and causing her depression. This low neurochemistry also made Valerie more passive, introverted, and mentally sluggish—all common characteristics of this type of depression.

After a while, Valerie's neurochemical configuration became her baseline; in other words, her brain began to recognize this arrangement of chemicals as normal. Similarly, the depression caused by this baseline became familiar to Valerie, and in an odd way, it seemed safe. This is the problem with the baseline and the familiar feelings it invokes: they are often regarded as safe even when they are uncomfortable, because the pain that is familiar is somehow less frightening than the pain that is unknown. For many people, depression is regarded as tolerable and even normal, at least for them.

No lecture from me was going to change Valerie's beliefs or her brain chemistry. For one thing, I don't possess a crystal ball, so I couldn't predict her future any better than she could. And if Valerie believed strongly enough that her marriage was doomed to fail, she could find a way to fulfill that belief, and her own prediction about the future would prove to have been the right one after all. Obviously, her belief system had to change. The question was, how could we change it?

I encouraged her to begin counseling as a way of examining her beliefs and creating a new set of goals and expectations about life. A qualified therapist could also help her work through the conflicts and pain she had experienced as a child. This process, of course, would take time and effort, and it was unlikely to have an immediate impact on her depression. Still, Valerie needed an ongoing support system to help her cope with her negative view of the future. Counseling could provide this support and would, in the long run, help change her behaviors, outlook, and brain chemistry.

Meanwhile, I put Valerie on a program that would change her brain chemistry in a relatively short period. This would help change her inner emotional condition, which in turn would help change her perceptions, interpretations, and beliefs about life.

Valerie's underlying brain-chemistry imbalance involved low levels of serotonin, dopamine, and norepinephrine. Valerie lacked self-esteem, confidence, and a sense of well-being, and her concentration was poor—all because of the low levels of serotonin. In fact, this deficiency was precisely why she had turned to alcohol and compulsive eating, especially sugar. Alcohol and sugar raise serotonin levels for short periods, but these elevations quickly fall off, and the net effect of such substances is a long-term deficiency in serotonin—and depression.

Valerie was also low in dopamine and norepinephrine, neurotransmitters associated with willpower, alertness, assertiveness, and aggression. When norepinephrine and dopamine are low, they also lead to depression, as well as loss of willpower and low energy, and these were all symptoms that Valerie exhibited.

This combination of low neurochemistry often makes it very difficult for people to face their difficulties squarely and take on new challenges. Many find it hard to leave the house. The world outside the front door is demanding, stimulating, and arousing. Driving to the supermarket in traffic will raise your norepinephrine and dopamine levels in minutes, along with your sense of stress and anxiety. Taking a job and struggling to meet the demands of employers and coworkers can send your norepinephrine and dopamine levels through the roof; again, your stress and anxiety levels will skyrocket, too. If your baseline brain chemistry considers these states normal and tolerable, you can function well under such conditions. But if your baseline says that such conditions are abnormal and intolerable, you'll retreat from these situations. Valerie could not bear stress or anxiety. The combination of low self-esteem and weak willpower made the challenges of the outside world seem overwhelming and frightening. Hence, she hid inside her home.

My approach was to increase her serotonin levels as quickly as possible and gradually increase norepinephrine. The first thing Valerie needed was foods and exercises that would create longer-lasting elevations in serotonin.

I explained how sugar and alcohol contribute to depression and strongly urged her to reduce significantly her intake of these substances and, if possible, eliminate them from her diet. At the same time, I had her gradually introduce foods that would promote slow increases in norepinephrine and dopamine, in order to restore her willpower and sense of inner strength.

I also provided a series of exercises that would reinforce these changes in brain chemistry. Finally, I suggested a variety of lifestyle factors, such as the types of music to listen to and the kinds of recreational activities to engage in, all of which would boost serotonin.

Valerie followed this program consistently but not perfectly. She had her lapses, as anyone would. Nevertheless, in a few months, she began to feel significantly better. The high-carbohydrate diet boosted serotonin and raised her self-esteem and sense of well-being significantly. At the same time, the protein-rich foods raised her levels of norepinephrine and dopamine. The exercise program strengthened her will and her sense of accomplishment. As she stuck to the exercise program, she increasingly felt that she could change for the better.

A year after Valerie began her program, she had lost a significant amount of weight; she had developed a far more open and supportive relationship with her husband; and she had an altogether new perspective on her life. She realized that she was not her mother and therefore did not have to repeat her mother's marriage nor her experience of life. She knew that she could make other choices that would provide her with very different experiences. Obviously, the counseling Valerie received gave her an important support system and did much to help her confront many long-standing beliefs. The brain-chemistry program, however, made it possible for her to change her beliefs, to take risks, and to improve her confidence, self-esteem, and sense of well-being in a relatively short period of time. Today, Valerie reports a complete recovery from chronic depression.

Valerie's is only one type of neurochemical imbalance that causes depression; this is the type I refer to as *"conditioned" Satiation* depression. I call her depression "conditioned" because it was the result of a family behavior pattern that she learned from one of her parents. I do not believe that Valerie inherited her depression; this would mean that her depression was part of her genetic makeup. None of Valerie's grandparents was depressed, as far as we could determine, nor were her aunts, uncles, and cousins. Rather, the depression emerged because the family was unable to reconcile an underlying conflict—that is, Valerie's parents were unable to confront and heal the reasons for their separation. Valerie's mother was clearly depressed. She had retreated from life into passivity and self-destructive behaviors. As I will explain in greater detail in the next two chapters, I call this a Satiation depression. I believe her father suffered from the opposite type, *Arousal* depression, meaning he was both depressed and anxious; like all Arousal types, he avoided feeling his depression by engaging in arousing activities—in his case, the high stress of his medical practice. He distracted himself from his own pain and that of his family by engaging in constant activity and maintaining a high degree of anxiety.

Valerie's mother was not anxious or driven. Instead, she sated and sedated herself to keep from feeling her pain, which nevertheless surfaced a lot of the time, only to be sedated again by alcohol or some other drug. Like her mother, Valerie herself was a Satiation-depressed person. This type is probably the most common, though Arousal depression—the combination of depression and anxiety—is also widespread. By knowing the type of depression a person suffers, I can offer an effective program that will address the underlying brain-chemistry imbalance.

Before I describe the different types of depression in greater detail, we must look more closely at brain chemistry and at how individual neurotransmitters affect our inner emotional and psychological state. Then we will be able to understand how these neurotransmitters can be brought back into balance to restore health.

Theories on the Cause of Depression

Clinical depression itself is as fundamental to the human experience as joy, laughter, and sadness. All of us experience feelings of loneliness, hopelessness, or melancholy from time to time. For most people, something inside them causes a rebound effect so that the "blues" don't hang on for very long. For reasons that are as mysterious as the laws that drive the weather, the depressed time passes, like a rainy night changing into a bright clear morning. Those who remain in the rainy night are said to suffer from clinical depression.

Clinical depression is more than merely an inner darkness. It is characterized by extreme sadness and anxiety, feelings of hopelessness and guilt, withdrawal from others, and loss of sleep, appetite, and sexual desire. Clinical depression is different in its intensity from the "down" feeling that all people experience at some point in their life. To a clinically depressed person, the feeling of helplessness is out of proportion to any external cause.

Traditionally, clinicians have categorized the causes of depression as *endogenous*, meaning it comes from within, and *exogenous*, meaning the cause of the depression comes from outside the body. Endogenous depression may be caused by an internal change in brain chemistry that was perhaps brought on by ongoing stress. With endogenous depression, a person cannot easily point to any single occurrence that may have triggered the condition. Rather, she has the feeling that she came to "the end of her rope" and simply gave up hope of overcoming the obstacles in her life. Exogenous depression is caused by some clear event or loss, such as the loss of one's job or the loss of a spouse. Such losses frequently bring on depression. The person's identity takes an enormous hit, and his understanding of who he is or what the purpose of his life may be often breaks down.

You may read about many different types of depression: exogenous, endogenous, unipolar, bipolar, manic-depressive, and others. But no matter what the diagnosis of the condition, the problem is the same—an out-of-balance brain chemistry.

Research is helping us understand that depression is some type of poor adaptation to stress. When we undergo stress, our endocrine system releases a group of hormones called *glucosteroids*, or "stress hormones," the most notable of which is cortisol. Scientists believe that secretions of high levels of cortisol may disrupt the balance and production of either serotonin or norepinephrine.

Thus, to paraphrase an old axiom, all roads lead to the neurotransmitters eventually. No matter what your diagnosis may be, the ultimate solution lies in reestablishing harmony in your brain chemistry. A psychiatrist may believe that restoring the neurochemical balance requires the use of one pharmaceutical agent or another. A psychologist may believe that the key is to change behaviors and maintain those changes over a long period of time until they become natural and comfortable. I believe that it means adopting certain behaviors and maintaining them consistently to restore harmony to brain chemistry rapidly. Unlike the psychiatrist, I do not rely on drugs, though I have recommended their use when I have believed they were necessary. Unlike the psychotherapist, I recommend changing behaviors that have less to do with a person's past than with the behaviors' effect on brain chemistry. I use powerful tools to change neurochemistry—namely, eating certain foods, performing certain exercises, adopting new behaviors, and thinking in new ways.

But unlike many physicians who believe that the cause of the condition is unimportant, I believe that a person's way of thinking and living is precisely what maintains the depression and makes it worse. This is because these behavioral factors help to maintain the person's current brain-chemistry imbalance.

Neurotransmitters: Powerful Droplets of Information

When I talk about brain chemistry, I'm talking, of course, about neurotransmitters. These are hormonelike chemicals that direct the workings of the central nervous system, including the brain, and thereby affect the entire body. Some neurotransmitters act as *catalysts:* they cause reactions or speed them up. Others are *inhibitors:* they slow down reactions or inhibit chemical events within the body.

Each of us experiences different rates of *neurotransmission* — that is, the speed of reactions within the nervous system and brain. We may experience fast thinking and quick physical reactions, for example, or slow thinking and slow physical reactions. Foods and behaviors that directly affect neurotransmitters can either speed up or slow down neurotransmission. For example, alcohol, as we all know, is a depressant and an inhibitor of the central nervous system. When you drink alcohol, your thoughts and physical reactions slow down. One of the ways alcohol slows neurotransmission is by temporarily boosting serotonin, which may slow neurotransmitters. If you drink enough alcohol, you'll slow down so much that you pass out.

Conversely, coffee and other caffeinated beverages and foods speed up neurotransmission, causing thoughts and reaction times to become much faster. Protein-rich foods also speed up neurotransmission, and they do it rapidly. Three ounces of fish, for example, will boost levels of dopamine and norepinephrine and cause neurotransmission to speed up in less than thirty minutes. So, too, will red meat, chicken, and eggs. As mentioned in Chapter One, dopamine and norepinephrine are both excitatory, or gas-pedal, brain chemicals. If your brain chemistry is dominated by excitatory neurotransmitters, neurotransmission will be too fast, and you will probably experience hyperactivity, erratic thinking, anxiety, and fear.

Dairy products are a mixture of protein and carbohydrate and therefore have less distinct effects on brain chemistry. Unlike many other animal foods, dairy products do contain carbohydrates, which boost serotonin, but the high protein content of milk and cheese mitigates the effects of carbohydrates. Thus, dairy foods fail to boost serotonin significantly.

While serotonin cannot be classified as either an inhibitor (brake) or an energizer (gas-pedal) chemical, it does affect neurotransmission.

When serotonin becomes too low, your thinking can become slow and dull. You will feel alone, isolated, unloved, and unworthy of love—a type of depression often referred to as "downer" depression. These same symptoms occur when the brain is dominated by *excesses* of the brake-pedal chemical GABA.

Inside your brain and muscles, brake-pedal and gas-pedal chemicals work in harmony, compensating for each other to create a balanced mental, emotional, and physical state. For example, dopamine—a gas-pedal chemical—and acetylcholine—a brake-pedal chemical—work together to coordinate muscle activity. Dopamine excites muscles and causes them to contract. Acetylcholine inhibits muscle activity, causing muscle activity to slow down. When the two are functioning properly, as they do for the vast majority of people, muscles move with perfect grace and precision. Every physical activity—whether it is walking, playing tennis or golf, driving your car, or making your bed—is made possible by the perfectly balanced interaction between dopamine and acetylcholine. Brake-pedal and gas-pedal neurochemicals are at work in virtually every physical and mental activity, including breathing, speech, sleep, and memory.

Let's examine more closely the three neurotransmitters that create depression—serotonin, dopamine, and norepinephrine—and look at how they can be altered to help us overcome it.

Serotonin: Peace, Concentration, and Well-Being

Research has consistently shown that low brain levels of serotonin are associated with mild to major depression, aggression, violence, and—for many—thoughts of suicide. In fact, low serotonin is probably the most common cause of depression. Consequently, many of the drugs used to treat depression, including the most popularly prescribed pharmaceuticals such as Prozac, work by making more serotonin available to brain cells.

The reason serotonin is so important to our mood and psychological health is that it is responsible for a whole host of positive feelings, including a sense of well-being, personal security, confidence, and higher levels of self-esteem. By raising the levels of serotonin, you increase your ability to relax and concentrate. Conversely, low serotonin is associated with confusion and the inability to concentrate.

Serotonin is essential for deep and restful sleep. All positive emotional conditions such as happiness and joy are associated with normal to elevated serotonin levels. Moderate to normal levels of serotonin are also associated with the absence of negative emotional states, such as anxiety, insecurity, anger, fear, and paranoia. In fact, serotonin may also affect how we experience pain. The more serotonin we have, the less pain we experience, and vice versa. There is a growing body of evidence showing that migraines may be associated with low serotonin and depression.

Feelings such as fear, anger, and paranoia are all associated with violence. Research conducted at the National Institutes of Mental Health (NIMH) has consistently shown that violent behavior is linked to low serotonin in both humans and animals. Studies have shown that military men with low serotonin are far more likely to have histories of violence and other forms of antisocial behavior. Moreover, the incidence of violence tends to increase among those with the lowest levels of serotonin. Other research has shown that men who commit suicide in particularly violent ways are low in serotonin.

Animal research confirms this pattern. Monkeys, for example, have well-structured societies in which each animal holds a certain place in the hierarchy; the animal's position in that hierarchy is a direct reflection of the amount of serotonin found in the animal's brain and nervous system. The leaders in monkey communities have the highest levels of serotonin—thus giving them the greatest sense of personal security and well-being—while those on the bottom rungs of the society have the lowest levels, thus making them most prone to insecurity, depression, violence, and other antisocial behaviors. These behaviors—

and the underlying brain chemistry that gives rise to them—are associated with low status and powerlessness within monkey society, just as they are within human society.

It is well established now that people who suffer from seasonal affective disorder (SAD) experience depression when deprived of adequate sunlight or other forms of full-spectrum lighting. In the absence of sunlight, the pineal gland produces higher levels of melatonin, a hormone that consumes serotonin. As more melatonin is produced, serotonin levels fall, thus giving rise to depression. When people with SAD are exposed to sufficient sunlight, melatonin levels decline, serotonin increases, and the depression disappears. Not surprisingly scientists have discovered that those with SAD also crave carbohydrates, a food that will promote the production of serotonin.

According to research conducted by Judith Wurtman, Ph.D., at the Massachusetts Institute of Technology (MIT), low serotonin is associated with the inability to control the amounts of food a person eats, as well as a reluctance to engage in consistent exercise. Not surprisingly, then, low serotonin is also associated with increases in weight. Wurtman reported in the *Journal of Affective Disorders* (October-November 1993) that when serotonin levels are restored, food intake is normalized and depression is diminished.

Interestingly, new research, reported in *Biological Psychiatry* (September 1, 1990), has discovered that eating disorders, such as bulimia and anorexia nervosa, are associated with low serotonin levels. Researchers have long noted the presence of depression among people with eating disorders. Studies have shown that binge eating, a symptom of bulimia, is caused by the brain's inability to absorb serotonin. This same inability, which leads to low levels of serotonin in the brain, may be a major cause of the depression associated with anorexia and other eating disorders.

Stress and the hormones it gives rise to—particularly catecholamines—may cause declines in serotonin, according to a study published in the *Journal of Clinical Psychiatry* (June 1991). Prolonged stress and high levels of stress hormones have long been known to create depression.

As we will see in the next three chapters, depression is associated with internal conflicts and the avoidance of events one believes will be difficult or challenging. According to a study reported in *International Clinical Psychopharmacology* (December 1991), people with normal serotonin levels worry less about impending adverse events and thus are more likely to confront difficult situations head on. Conversely, those with low serotonin have more anxiety over impending adverse events and also have a far greater tendency to avoid events that they expect will be difficult. The choice between facing a difficult situation or fleeing from it, scientists now believe, may well depend on serotonin levels. In any case, a breakdown in the *serotonergic pathway*— as the cells that depend on serotonin are called—is now believed to be associated both with avoidance behaviors and with the depression that so often accompanies them.

Low Levels of Serotonin

People with low levels of serotonin experience

- Declines in mood
- Depression
- Low energy and fatigue
- Low self-esteem
- Poor concentration
- Confusion
- Difficulty making decisions
- Fluctuations in appetite (such as cravings for carbohydrates, combined with little appetite for other foods)
- Decreased sex drive
- Excessive feelings of guilt and unworthiness

Consistently low serotonin, as we have already seen, can lead to violence, antisocial behavior, and even suicide.

Boosting Serotonin Levels

Interestingly, very few people today have naturally high serotonin levels. This may be the result of the mental, emotional, and physical stress of modern daily life, since such stress diminishes serotonin levels.

Prozac and other similar drugs all work by increasing the amounts of serotonin at the synapse—the tiny gap between nerve cells, or neurons. By increasing the availability of serotonin, these drugs eliminate many negative emotions, boost self-esteem and confidence, and very often encourage people to express themselves in ways that they previously felt were impossible. Unfortunately, these drugs have extensive side effects, as I pointed out in Chapter One, and rarely if ever do they have exclusively positive effects on people. The side effects include increased depression, anxiety, nervous tension, insomnia, drowsiness, tremors, sweating, gastrointestinal distress, nausea, diarrhea, dizziness, and light-headedness. The increase in depression may be paradoxical or may occur because the drug affected the wrong brain chemical.

Boosting Serotonin Levels Naturally

Positive thoughts and emotions boost serotonin levels in the brain, just as anxiety-ridden thoughts and fear increase dopamine and norepinephrine. Thus, we are all changing our brain chemistries constantly, whether we are depressed or in fine spirits. So one of the ways to escape depression is to understand which behaviors promote serotonin and which ones diminish this all-important neurotransmitter. Among the most powerful ways to increase serotonin are certain types of foods, exercises, music, and lifestyle factors such as meditation and prayer.

Let's take a closer look.

FOODS THAT INCREASE SEROTONIN AND DIMINISH DEPRESSION

Depression consistently has been shown to trigger increases in appetite and cravings for carbohydrate-rich foods and chocolate. So, too, have feelings of being rejected, which of course is a fundamental part of the experience of depression for most people. One of the most common responses to feelings of rejection or failure is to eat something sweet as a way of reducing the pain we feel. We have such cravings because most forms of carbohydrates—from whole grains to refined sugars and sweets—increase brain levels of serotonin, and they do it rapidly. As we all know, we can change our brain chemistry in a matter of minutes simply by eating a carbohydrate-rich food. Once we've eaten that chocolate éclair or jelly doughnut or ice cream sundae, the world seems a little less bleak, even if not altogether right. This is one of the reasons bakery items and ice cream continue to be so popular—because carbohydrates and sweet foods are so effective at medicating our moods.

Carbohydrates increase blood levels of tryptophan, an amino acid that acts as a precursor to serotonin. When you eat a carbohydrate-rich food, your blood fills up with tryptophan, which in turn produces lots of serotonin in your brain.

Most animal foods, such as red meats, contain tryptophan, but they also contain a wide assortment of other amino acids. All of these amino acids compete with each other to get past the blood-brain barrier and thus into your brain. The transport system that carries amino acids into the brain allows only a restricted number of amino acids to pass through. Each of the amino acids in animal proteins competes with the others for a seat on the transport system. In the end, less tryptophan actually gets into the brain's chemistry and consequently less serotonin is produced. The net effect is that the more red meat and other animal foods you eat, the less serotonin you produce.

There are two types of carbohydrates—*complex* and *refined*. Complex carbohydrates are sugar molecules that are bound together in fiber and must be digested in the small intestine in order to release the sugar into the blood. Digestion tends to be slow and methodical.

Consequently, the sugars are released into the bloodstream in a slow and steady flow. This means that complex carbohydrates, found in whole grains, fresh vegetables, and fruits, tend to provide a long-lasting flow of energy and tryptophan to the blood and brain.

Refined carbohydrates are simple sugars that have been stripped of their fiber and nutrition during food processing. The sugars have been released from the foods they originally came in and then added to other foods, such as doughnuts, cakes, and candy. These simple sugars do not need digestion. Rather, they enter your bloodstream directly from your mouth. They also make their way into the bloodstream through the small intestine but without the long process of digestion. Consequently, your blood sugar rises instantly, causing an initial burst of tryptophan and serotonin. However, the body burns off this abundance of sugar as quickly as it absorbs it, causing a condition often referred to as *hypoglycemia*, or low blood sugar. When blood-sugar levels are low, there's little tryptophan left in the blood, and serotonin levels drop off. Hence, many people with hypoglycemia complain of fatigue and depression. They also become addicted to refined or simple sugars, bingeing constantly on cakes, candy, sodas, and other sources of simple sugars. Thus, their blood sugar rises and falls rapidly, leaving them in a constant state of craving yet also feeling weak and depressed.

Some people who are depressed turn to drugs to create even stronger serotonin responses. Among the most popular drugs that increase serotonin are alcohol and marijuana. Both of these drugs will boost brain levels of serotonin, but both have negative side effects, especially in the young because they create such extreme reactions in brain chemistry. These side effects are well documented in alcohol abuse. Now, new research is showing that regular marijuana use weakens the ability of the brain to concentrate, recall facts, and solve problems. And long-term use, science is showing, significantly slows neurotransmission, causing the brain to become dull and forgetful.

The most effective foods for boosting serotonin and maintaining a healthy brain chemistry are those that are rich in carbohydrates. (You'll find a complete list of these foods in Chapter Seven.)

EXERCISES THAT BOOST SEROTONIN AND DIMINISH DEPRESSION

All relaxing forms of exercise are serotonin boosters. (These exercises are listed in Chapter Seven.) I particularly recommend spending time in nature. Take walks in the park or the forest and enjoy the peace and tranquillity of the trees, a river, or a pond. Walk on the beach and listen to the rhythms of the waves. Let the ocean lap against your feet and take your mind to the distant horizon. In a strict sense, walking in the forest or on the beach is exercise, but because it also stills your mind, you hardly realize that your body is being active. Other recommendations include freshwater or saltwater fishing. Learn to fly cast or use a spinning reel. As a fisherman once told me, "Fishing is guaranteed peace of mind. No matter what your problems are, they seem to vanish on the banks of a river."

Such experiences create a peaceful mind in large part because they boost serotonin. In fact, they involve us in a positive cycle: the settings themselves are peaceful and induce us to relax, which is serotonin boosting. And these higher levels of serotonin inspire thoughts that are positive and relaxing, which in turn boost serotonin again.

ACTIVITIES, THOUGHTS, AND FEELINGS THAT BOOST SEROTONIN

Indeed, all peaceful thoughts and feelings and their catalysts are serotonin boosters. Scientists have even found that placebos—pills that have no actual biochemical value—often are just as powerful in improving a person's state of mind as anti-depressant drugs. As researchers noted in the medical journal *Drugs* (Supplement 43, 2:32–37, 1992), "several investigators have observed high placebo response rates, and in some studies there has been a similar response rate to imipramine and placebo treatment." The reason placebos can be so powerful at overcoming depression is that people *believe* they are getting a drug that will change their brain chemistries. This belief alone is enough to affect their brain chemistry positively, changing it sufficiently to reduce and even overcome depression.

Among the most effective tools for boosting serotonin are reading (especially inspirational literature), prayer, and meditation. Positive imaging routines that induce deep relaxation can be powerful ways to increase serotonin, as well.

Another way to increase serotonin—one that all of us have experienced—is to listen to peaceful, gentle music, such as folk, soft jazz, rhythm and blues, and various show tunes and classical pieces, especially some of the works of Bach, Brahms, Chopin, Handel, and Haydn. *Madame Butterfly* and many other operas are serotonin boosters. Though opera includes a lot of loud and emotional singing, it is also deeply moving and highly cathartic.

What these musical works have in common is their ability to open us up to inspiring feelings. These feelings awaken us to the beauty of life. They can also put us in touch with our pain, which can be very healing, especially if this helps us release negative emotions. Feelings of anger, bitterness, betrayal, and loss often block the conscious mind from the deeper realms of forgiveness, gratitude, and love. Great music has an uncanny way of putting us in touch with both the pain and the beauty of life. It allows us to experience grief and sadness, yet it helps us to transcend it and achieve deeper insight and inner peace. This transcendence is a powerful serotonin booster.

Finally, service to others and finding a sense of purpose in the larger community are also serotonin boosters. Why? Because such work gives us a sense of security and linkage to others. We are all social beings, and we yearn to find a place in society where we can feel useful and fulfilled. This is why so many depressed people who decide to do some type of social work or volunteerism find themselves overcoming their depression.

Dopamine: Alertness, Energy, and Aggression

As with serotonin, deficient amounts of dopamine are also responsible for depression but for very different reasons. Dopamine gives us a sense of strength, vitality, energy, and personal power. Consequently, those who are deficient in dopamine often suffer from lethargy, weakness, and a kind of vegetative depression.

On the other hand, too much dopamine can lead to anxiety, fear, excessive nervous tension, paranoia, and delusion. The anxiety produced by excess dopamine—and its derivative neurotransmitter, norepinephrine—can cover an underlying depression. (We'll look further at this pattern in the next chapter.)

The production of dopamine in the central nervous system and brain triggers a whole host of physical, mental, and emotional reactions, all related to heightened states of alertness, aggression, mental and physical agility, and greater problem-solving skills. Dopamine production is increased—sometimes rapidly—whenever we confront a challenging mental or physical problem or a threatening situation, including being in an argument, being stopped by a police car, or being criticized by someone in authority. Dopamine is also increased in anticipation of, and during, an exciting activity, such as sex, a sporting event, a debate, or any type of competitive situation.

In all of these situations, dopamine speeds up the transmission of nerve impulses from one neuron to the next, making thoughts and physical reactions faster and often more precise. With heightened amounts of dopamine, the brain works quickly to solves problems. We think, speak, and breathe more rapidly. Heart rate increases instantly. Muscle coordination is optimized, giving us greater physical agility and the power to run faster, jump higher, and move with more power. Dopamine is also responsible for giving us more energy. The moment you are confronted with a competitive or threatening situation, dopamine gives you the energy needed to deal with that situation.

Dopamine is essential for all muscle activity, which means that it is essential to every type of physical activity in which we engage. Just as dopamine is essential for muscle activity, it is also depleted the longer muscles work. Thus, all strenuous, exciting, and arousing physical acts leave us lower in dopamine than when we began that activity. The result is that we feel more relaxed and peaceful after exercise than before it.

Dopamine is elevated with the use of certain recreational drugs, especially cocaine. By immediately increasing dopamine, cocaine causes temporary bursts of energy and euphoria, and short but intense periods of clarity and mental acuity. The mind is pushed to work at its optimal limits, which makes it extremely fast at problem solving. The person on cocaine often talks and gestures rapidly, cannot sit still, and experiences inordinate amounts of energy—at least until she crashes. At that point, delusional thinking, paranoia, and fears set in. As with other addictive drugs, cocaine inevitably has an opposite effect on the brain, by depleting the body of dopamine and causing lower baseline dopamine levels, as well as depression, confusion, withdrawal, the need for sleep, and a craving for more cocaine.

Dopamine and Norepinephrine

Dopamine is a building block in the creation of norepinephrine, another excitatory neurotransmitter that is especially important in the onset and treatment of depression. Three chemicals—dopamine, norepinephrine, and adrenaline, a by-product of dopamine—make possible the "fight-or-flight" reactions of the brain and body. Thus, all responses involving fear and increased cardiovascular, respiratory, and muscle activity depend on heightened levels of dopamine and norepinephrine. Together, dopamine and norepinephrine and the cells involved in their transmission are referred to as the *noradrenergic pathway* within the brain.

As excitatory neurotransmitters, dopamine and norepinephrine give us instant energy and arousal. When one or both of these chemicals are deficient in the brain and nervous system, you feel tired, lethargic, fatigued. If either of these becomes severely restricted, you become depressed and vegetative. People with depression resulting from low dopamine or low norepinephrine often say, "I don't have the energy I need to confront my problems. The minute I think about my problems, I get weak and tired. I can't think about doing anything to solve my problems."

The pathway that handles norepinephrine and dopamine transmission is the energy pathway. If you are deficient in norepinephrine or dopamine, you probably experience chronic lethargy and require more sleep, yet your mind may seem to function normally. Your mental capacity is intact, and you are unaware of any memory impairment. Your only serious complaint will be similar to that expressed by sufferers of chronic fatigue syndrome (CFS). (I am convinced that many people have been diagnosed with CFS when they're actually depressed.)

Valerie, in the example cited at the beginning of this chapter, suffered from low serotonin and low dopamine and norepinephrine. This combination made her both depressed and fatigued. Many depressed people have low serotonin but normal dopamine and norepinephrine, which means that they are depressed, but they have the energy to do their jobs. My questionnaire (see Chapter Three and the survey at the end of the book) asks people a series of questions that help determine whether the person is simply depressed or depressed and chronically lethargic. You will be asked to fill out one of these questionnaires in the next chapter to determine whether you are a Satiation-depressed or an Arousal-depressed person.

In summary, the depression associated with low dopamine or low norepinephrine is much more vegetative and lethargic than the depression associated with low serotonin alone.

Distinguishing Between Imbalanced Dopamine and Imbalanced Norepinephrine

Imbalances in dopamine tend to affect the psyche and create disturbances in perception—including hallucinations—more than do imbalances in norepinephrine. People with excessively low or excessively high dopamine tend to have great difficulty perceiving life accurately. The main difference between the two extremes of dopamine is that low dopamine is usually associated with low energy, withdrawal from life, and thoughts of suicide, while high dopamine is associated with high energy, paranoia, and violence, often directed toward oneself. Balanced levels of dopamine are essential for healthy perceptions of reality.

Elevated Dopamine Levels

When mildly elevated, dopamine increases

- Arousal
- Awareness and alertness
- Assertiveness
- Aggression
- Respiration, cardiovascular, and muscle activity

Moderately elevated dopamine levels can lead to

- Anxiety (consistent elevations can lead to chronic anxiety)
- Fear
- Feelings of detachment
- Excessive energy
- Sleep disturbances
- Increased sex drive

Excessive dopamine that remains chronically high can lead to

- Delusions
- Hallucinations
- Inappropriate responses and affect
- Paranoia
- Social isolation
- Schizophrenia
- Psychosis

Low Dopamine Levels

A deficiency in dopamine can cause

- Depression
- Low energy
- Muscular disturbances and Parkinson's disease

- Need for excess sleep
- Withdrawal
- Suicide or preoccupation with thoughts of suicide

Boosting Dopamine Levels

Many of the older anti-depressant medications affected both serotonin and dopamine. Wellbutrin is a newer anti-depressant that has more specific effects on norepinephrine and dopamine. The amphetamines, which fell into disfavor because of their addictive properties, increase dopamine and norepinephrine levels. They can be very effective with certain individuals who have only dopamine or norepinephrine deficiencies. Ritalin is also often used successfully for these individuals.

Boosting Dopamine Levels Naturally

FOODS THAT INCREASE DOPAMINE

All foods containing protein increase blood levels of the amino acid tyrosine, which is converted into dopamine in the brain. Chapter Seven provides complete lists of the foods richest in protein; some of the healthiest examples include fish, chicken eaten without the skin, and a wide variety of beans.

How much protein do you need to promote an arousal response?

Three to four ounces of a protein-rich food, such as a piece of fish the size of a deck of cards, will elevate dopamine levels and change your mood and brain function significantly in less than ten minutes. You will think more rapidly and clearly after a high-protein meal. You will also have more energy and will be more alert, assertive, and aggressive toward a particular problem. You will not be able to concentrate for very long, however, nor are you likely to be able to sit still. To relax and concentrate, you need serotonin-boosting foods—namely, carbohydrates.

If you want the effects of a dopamine-boosting meal, do not combine protein and carbohydrates, because the carbohydrates will mitigate the effects of the protein on the brain. The carbohydrates will slow down brain function and make you more relaxed, focused, and passive. More than likely, you will want to sit still for a while and think things over—in other words, you'll experience the exact opposite of the dopamine-elevated consciousness.

EXERCISES THAT BOOST DOPAMINE

All strenuous exercise and competitive situations—including sports, video games, and board games such as chess—will increase dopamine rapidly and thus create feelings of alertness, enhance clarity of mind, and produce heightened anxiety. Exercise, whether it involves competition or not, drives up dopamine, but it also burns it off in muscle activity, leaving you feeling physically, mentally, and emotionally relieved afterward. It is true that highly competitive people may feel bad after they lose a game, but the physical exertion of playing will have left them relaxed and maybe even exhausted. Very often, the combatants in a sporting event—such as boxing, football, tennis, or basketball—speak highly of each other after the game is over and embrace as they leave the field. This reflects the fact that their brain chemistries are very different after the game than they were before it. Dopamine is no longer rushing through their veins and brains, creating the aggression and fear that they experienced before the game. In its place is serotonin, which elevates in the aftermath of physical exertion to create feelings of well-being, relaxation, and peace.

These feelings of relief, accomplishment, and relaxation are also related to an increase in endorphins. Endorphins are morphinelike compounds in your brain that are released to relieve pain and reward you for doing something that your body recognizes as especially good for you, such as exercise. The brain secretes beta endorphins after twenty minutes of running or performing some other aerobic exercise. This is what causes the "natural high" that runners often refer to.

Numerous studies, among them a study published in the *International Journal of Obesity* (5:57, 1981), have shown that exercise alleviates depression. Another study examined the effects of exercise on patients in psychiatric hospitals and found that exercise significantly decreased depression and anxiety, and increased a sense of accomplishment.

The problem with video games, on the other hand, is that they not only create tremendous arousal, increasing levels of dopamine and norepinephrine in the brain and levels of adrenaline in the blood, but they also require little or no physical exertion. This means that the increased levels of dopamine, norepinephrine, and adrenaline are not fully utilized during the game. Very often people who have played a video game walk away feeling nervous, tense, and irritable. Their hands and legs literally shake. If they were to go out for a run, they would burn off the gas-pedal chemicals and feel fine again, but usually they try to reduce the stress caused by the excitement by eating or drinking foods that are rich in sugar (a form of carbohydrate, as we've seen). This lowers dopamine and norepinephrine and increases serotonin, allowing them some peace of mind and physical relaxation. They are literally medicating themselves with sugar in order to deal with the anxiety created by the dopamine. Yet the dopamine never really leaves the tissues and is simply waiting until some other form of arousal stimulates another round of excitement, anxiety, and stress. Many people—especially the young—are continually bouncing back and forth between arousal and satiation, between the "fight-or-flight" response and the dreamy world of sugar- or drug-induced satiation. These heightened states of arousal and their concomitant levels of dopamine make dependence on sugar, refined foods, and drugs extremely tempting.

ACTIVITIES, THOUGHTS, AND FEELINGS THAT INCREASE DOPAMINE

All images, music, and activities that are exciting and arousing increase dopamine and norepinephrine. Dancing, action movies, rock music, musical theater, and exciting classical music, such as the music of Beethoven, are all arousing and thus increase these neurotransmitters. Virtually any action-packed movie is dopamine producing. A carnival, a fair, or the circus is a highly arousing event. A ride on a roller coaster or a Ferris wheel is a huge dopamine producer. Often, just walking along a busy street in a major city is arousing.

You can increase both dopamine and norepinephrine simply by thinking about something exciting or allowing yourself the anticipation of some pleasurable form of excitement. All thoughts and images of an upcoming pleasurable event increase dopamine. Unfortunately, so too do expectations of adverse events. And therein lies a big problem for those who are low in dopamine: they associate all forms of arousal with negative consequences and therefore retreat into safe havens that contribute to their depression.

Many people who are shut-ins and depressed are locked into an unfortunate cycle in which all expectations of arousal trigger anxiety. Consequently, they retreat from arousing situations out of fear. They don't realize that they are locked into a restricted world by the images in their minds and the brain chemistry that such images create. They have become intolerant of any increase in dopamine.

Many people who are deficient in dopamine believe themselves to be weak and incapable of dealing with stressful situations. They fear such situations and try to control their lives to avoid all forms of stress. Even if you describe the perfect outing in which all events will be pleasurable and fun, such people worry that something will go wrong. They know that they will not be able to control the event, and any event that is out of their control is terrifying. Thus, they retreat from all situations that have the potential to create anxiety and fear. But this retreat robs them of the joy of living and thus leads inevitably to depression.

In order to raise dopamine gradually and bring joy into their lives, those who are low in this neurotransmitter must start to experience and enjoy arousing situations in small doses. In effect, they must challenge themselves by taking small steps toward situations that will raise their dopamine levels. For some, this may mean little more than a couple of hours at the shopping mall or a night at the movies. For others, it may mean dining out and dancing or listening to music that is arousing. Only the depressed individuals will know what their limits are and what is an appropriate challenge for them. Yet each time they engage in a pleasurable arousing activity, they will find their depression lessening a bit. If they continue to have enjoyable dopamine-producing experiences, they will gradually change their baseline brain chemistries and restore balance and harmony to their lives.

Norepinephrine: Speeding Up Your Thoughts

When brain chemistry is low in norepinephrine, depression is often the result. If norepinephrine gets too low, it can cause the low-energy, or vegetative, type of depression, along with feelings of powerlessness and insecurity. Like dopamine, norepinephrine can be increased naturally and with little effort.

Norepinephrine is essential to all muscle activity, to the constriction and dilation of blood vessels, and to the opening of bronchioles in the respiratory tract. It elevates the heart rate and creates heightened states of awareness, alertness, and assertiveness. Normal levels give us the ability to react quickly and aggressively to demanding situations and to danger. They also give us a strong sense of willpower. Like dopamine, norepinephrine increases the rate of neurotransmission, or the speed of your thoughts.

Low Norepinephrine Levels

The symptoms of low norepinephrine levels include

- Depression
- Low energy
- Weight gain
- Changes in menstruation
- Decreased sex drive

Chronically low norepinephrine can manifest as

- Chronic, severe depression
- Short-term memory loss
- Dull or slow thought processes
- Male impotence

High Levels of Norepinephrine

Excess norepinephrine causes

- Insomnia
- Hallucinations
- Attention deficit disorder
- Excessive energy
- Elevated heart rate
- Increased blood pressure
- Rapid breathing
- Weight loss
- Increased sex drive
- Disorientation

Boosting Norepinephrine Levels Through Drugs

Many anti-depressant drugs are designed to increase norepinephrine. Among these are the monoamine oxidase inhibitors, such as Nardil. These often result in symptoms that are typical of excessively high norepinephrine, including weight loss, anxiety, and phobias.

Boosting Norepinephrine Levels Naturally

FOODS THAT INCREASE NOREPINEPHRINE

Protein-rich foods increase tyrosine, which in turn boosts norepinephrine. Thus, all the protein-rich foods listed in Chapter Seven will increase norepinephrine. Among the healthiest of these are low-fat fish, beans, chicken, and turkey. Red meat and eggs will also boost norepinephrine levels significantly, but their fat and cholesterol contents decrease their health benefits.

EXERCISES AND LIFESTYLE FACTORS THAT BOOST NOREPINEPHRINE
The same exercises and lifestyle factors that raise dopamine will also increase brain levels of norepinephrine.

How Neurotransmitters Become Imbalanced

In general, there are three ways that neurotransmitters become imbalanced and create the basis for depression:

Through a genetic disorder passed down to us from our parents and grandparents

Through conditioning or learned patterns from our families

Through some kind of stressful situation or traumatic event

Any one of these situations can establish a baseline neurochemistry that supports depression. I call the first of these three *genetic* or *inherited;* the second, *generational* or *conditioned;* and the third, *situational.* There can also be some combination of these—a learned pattern might lead to a mild, chronic depression that can be exacerbated by a divorce or the loss of a job, for example. This could result in an even deeper and more severe condition.

What is especially important to keep in mind is that to varying degrees, our baseline neurochemistry determines what we believe to be true, and these beliefs are highly subjective. Yet at the same time, this subjective view of life is supporting our brain chemistry and thus the depression itself. It isn't just that the brain chemistry is imbalanced, as if this were a separate subject on its own, but that this imbalance may be causing us to see the world in dark and negative terms. Brain chemistry is the basis for our subjective outlook, and this outlook in turn supports the brain chemistry. We must break the cycle if healing is to take place.

Genetic or Inherited Depression

Imbalances in brain chemistry can be passed down from one or both parents to their children via their genes, causing a tendency toward depression. There is also a range of inherited diseases that can lead to depression, such as hypothyroidism, diabetes, hypoadrenalism, parathyroidism, and other illnesses.

Each of these illnesses affects our brain chemistry by altering some part of our hormonal system. For example, parathyroidism, hypoadrenalism, or hypothyroidism may cause a reduction in serotonin or dopamine, while hyperadrenalism may cause an increase in dopamine.

Like all other depressions, genetically based depressions alter one's perceptions and beliefs. Inherited depression can lead to compulsive behaviors, including perfectionism and various types of addictions, such as alcoholism, gambling, and drug abuse. But genetically influenced depressions can be managed with appropriate changes in lifestyle and nutrition—the kinds of programs I offer in Part Two of this book.

As I will show in the next three chapters, all forms of depression can be broadly categorized into two types—downer depression, or what I call Satiation depression, and anxious depression, or what I call Arousal depression. Depressions that stem from genetically based imbalances are no different; they, too, turn out to be either Satiation or Arousal depressions.

The genetically based Satiation depression occurs when there is low serotonin and low norepinephrine and dopamine. Such low neurochemistry can occur for any one of several reasons, including the insufficient production of neurotransmitters or the premature breakdown of a neurochemical before it has its normal effect. Whatever the cause, the person does not have enough neurotransmission to feel normal. This deficiency can cause misperceptions, misinterpretations, and even false beliefs, especially about himself. In the Satiation-depressed person, the imbalance causes introversion and a retreat from the stimuli of daily events and situations. Compulsive behavioral disorders can also set in, such as perfectionism and ritualistic behaviors. People with genetically based Satiation depression tend to be passive, and they search for ways to escape all intense or demanding situations, since these would drive up dopamine and norepinephrine and create an unbearable tension and anxiety.

Inherited depression can also lead to a combination of depression and anxiety, or what I call Arousal depression. In this case, there may be low serotonin along with abnormally high levels of norepinephrine and/or dopamine. People who suffer from Arousal depression are far more aware of their chronic anxiety, which drives their behavior, than of the deep and painful depression that lies beneath the anxiety. Many people who are both anxious and depressed try to maintain a lifestyle that will prevent them from feeling their depression. They eat lots of protein, drink lots of coffee, and maintain a high level of stress in their life. All of these behaviors keep dopamine and norepinephrine levels up, which masks the underlying low serotonin and its consequent depression.

People with genetically based depression can usually identify a parent—or both parents—who was depressed. The parents may have covered their depression with anxiety, compulsive behaviors, or addictions, but beneath the nervous tension, the frenzy for housecleaning, the boredom, the alcohol, or the drugs lay a depression that drove Mother or Father. Very often, a grandparent or both grandparents were also depressed. With some effort, children of depressed parents can identify depression as a characteristic that runs through the family.

It's hard for a genetically based depressed person—no matter whether she is a Satiation type or an Arousal type—to overcome her depression with psychotherapy alone. This is because the neurochemical baseline has been established and reinforced by both genetic and behavioral factors. Often the behaviors have been in place for so long—usually since childhood—that it is difficult for the person to choose to act differently, at least until her brain chemistry has changed.

The best way to treat genetically based depressions is to work with the brain chemistry first and then go into the person's psychology.

Anti-depressants tend to work well in these cases because they change the underlying brain chemistry immediately, and this in turn allows genetically depressed people to perceive themselves and the world around them differently.

For those whose depressions are genetically based and who have contemplated suicide, drug therapy is often essential; I encourage everyone who has a family pattern of depression and who has entertained self-destructive thoughts to see a physician immediately. Part Two of this book offers a program for the Satiation-depressed person and one for the Arousal-depressed person; these programs work well for genetically based depression. They can be used along with your physician's treatments or independently, if your doctor does not recommend drugs.

In Chapter Six, I describe situations that can reinforce or plunge a person deeper into depression. These situations, which I call triggers, plunge us into emotional crisis, feelings of low self-worth, or fear. The genetically depressed person must become aware of his triggers in order to take preventive steps, which include following the program to sustain higher serotonin levels, as described in Part Two.

The following self-test can help you determine if you suffer from a genetically influenced depression.

➤ Self-Test for Genetically Based Depression

1. Does/did your biological father have depressions?

2. Does/did your biological mother have depressions?

3. Do/did two or more of your biological grandparents show signs of depression?

4. Do/did two or more of your biological siblings show signs of depression?

5. Does/did one or more of your biological children show signs of depression?

TOTAL YES _____   TOTAL NO _____

"Yes" answers to two or more questions indicate a possible genetic influence in your depression. If you have four or more "yes" answers, your genes play a primary influence in your depression. Your recovery will certainly require manipulation of your neurochemistry in order to overcome your depression. I recommend that you see a physician and at the same time follow the program best suited to your condition, as described in the next three chapters.

Generational or Conditioned

All families have patterns of behavior that help to determine the brain chemistry of family members. Acute behavioral disorders within families can give rise to extreme brain-chemistry imbalances. Physical abuse of children is a good example.

Ronald, a former client of mine, was raised by alcoholic parents who routinely erupted into rage and physical violence. Out of the blue, Ronald's mother or father would become angry and start hitting him for some trumped-up reason. He was a target and an outlet for their rage. These conditions shaped Ronald's brain chemistry, making him exceedingly high in dopamine and norepinephrine, two chemicals that kept him on red alert at all times. At the same time, he was low in serotonin, which gave him low self-esteem, sleep disturbances, and a sense of despair about his future. Ronald emerged from his family anxious and depressed, though for most of his childhood and adult years he didn't know he was depressed. All he could experience were his anxiety, nervousness, and fear, which existed like a wall of tension hiding an underlying pain. When I first started to work with Ronald, his primary goal was to reduce his anxiety. But as we diminished the nervous tension, he began to feel the emptiness beneath it. He would deal with that emptiness by filling his life up with work-related pressures and deadlines. This distracted him from the pain that existed below the stress, but he rarely if ever experienced any sort of satisfaction from his life or his accomplishments.

Gradually, we were able to get his serotonin levels up and decrease his dopamine levels by changing his diet and getting him to exercise regularly. With the gradual increase in serotonin and decrease in dopamine, he began to sleep better, his confidence increased, and he felt better about himself. Remarkably, these feelings formed a foundation that allowed him to seek counseling and start to explore his inner issues. Ronald's story demonstrated that the core issues of our lives do not go away simply by changing the brain chemistry. On the contrary, an improvement in brain chemistry can give us some basis for *dealing* with those issues. By changing his lifestyle and confronting his inner pain, Ronald was able to make a fundamental change in his baseline neurochemistry; in short, he experienced a physical, emotional, and spiritual transformation.

Ronald's story illustrates only one type of dysfunction that confronts families and especially children. Verbal, emotional, and sexual abuse can cause extreme imbalances in brain chemistry similar to and even worse than Ronald's. Many children are raised by parents who feel powerless and engage in all kinds of deceits in order to avoid dealing directly with their problems. Powerlessness often gives rise to low serotonin and low norepinephrine, since the belief that we can do nothing creates feelings of inertia, lethargy, and despair; all of these diminish norepinephrine levels. This makes us feel as if there's no way we can get past the big wall that rises in front of us. All the emotional, intellectual, and psychological benefits of norepinephrine—such as willpower and determination—are dampened and dissipated. We simply stop believing in ourselves. Such a sense of powerlessness also creates low self-esteem and fear. Taken together, these feelings can lead to depression.

On the other side of the coin is the family who does too much and who never stops to experience intimacy. Norepinephrine and dopamine are skyrocketing, while serotonin levels are low. Such behaviors frequently give rise to overachievers. People stake their entire identity and self-worth on achievement. Many overachievers, who are also sometimes called "type A" personalities, are depressed, but they don't know it until they face a life crisis, frequently in midlife. They lose their jobs, or experience a divorce, or undergo a health crisis, and suddenly they're depressed. What they didn't know is that they were depressed all along; they were simply masking that depression with the drive to achieve.

Perfectionism and many forms of compulsive behaviors are related to these kinds of family patterns and the brain chemistries that are altered before adulthood, such as genetic, inherited, or generational influences. Perfectionism leads to overachieving and, in all too many cases, to suicide. Recent studies have examined the relationship between overachievers and self-destructive thinking. What scientists are finding is that perfectionism is often a compensation for those who are extremely sensitive to criticism and have exceedingly low self-esteem. These symptoms suggest very low levels of serotonin and high levels of dopamine and norepinephrine. This can be a dangerous combination for many people, because the high dopamine can lead to delusion and hostility that is turned against themselves.

As I said earlier, all kinds of depression can be divided into Satiation and Arousal types. Ronald was an Arousal-depressed person, with high norepinephrine and low serotonin.

As with inherited or genetically based depression, people with conditioned depression must also be aware of trigger situations that remind them of old events or patterns in their families and that lower their self-esteem, bring on painful memories, or plunge them into despair or fear. Chapter Six will help you become aware of these trigger situations, and the programs described in Part Two will help change your brain chemistry so that you can cope with them adequately.

Situational Causes

Situational causes of depression may consist of abrupt traumas and changes in life, such as the sudden loss of a loved one or of a job or the sudden onset of an illness; they can also arise from ongoing problems in a relationship or in the individual, such as unresolved anger, perfectionism, or workaholism.

The loss of a loved one is one of the most painful events that life offers. For those who have lost a spouse or someone with whom they were bonded for many years, the loss can feel as if part of themselves has died. Many who experience such a loss question whether or not to go on living, and it is not an easy question to answer. For many, the decision to continue to live brings with it tremendous guilt; going on with life may feel like a betrayal of the loved one who is gone. Once we decide to go on, however, we must deal with the ongoing pain that transforms even the most mundane of situations. These feelings, which are natural and even inescapable, all cause a diminution of serotonin, which in turn causes a whole host of emotional and psychological disturbances that can lead to depression. In addition, the overwhelming sense of injustice at having someone we love taken away from us triggers tremendous anger and frustration. These feelings, in turn, increase stress and brain levels of dopamine and norepinephrine. For many, this hostility goes unexpressed and is turned inward, causing self-hatred and self-destructive behaviors.

Another type of loss is divorce, which can bring very different kinds of emotions than those associated with the death of a loved one. In divorce, both partners suffer a loss, but in most cases one of them precipitates the separation, which means that the other usually suffers a greater sense of loss and betrayal. Divorced people can feel a loss of self-esteem, confidence, and inner peace, often due to the alterations in brain chemistry caused by the loss.

Often, intense stress that suddenly stops can result in depression. Let's say that you experience a lot of stress around the holidays. You feel pressured to make everything right for others, so you purchase gifts, spend a lot of money, and run around like a crazy person for weeks prior to the big day. All of this, of course, raises norepinephrine levels dramatically, causing anxiety, stress, and even fear that all will not go right. Your norepinephrine levels can get so high that the mental and physical tension can become unbearable. One day, you suddenly shut down and decide you're not doing any more. Or the stress continues right up to the holiday itself. The event culminates either with joy or sadness or anger, and suddenly it is over. In either of these cases, there has been a sudden shift in brain chemistry. For weeks you have been maintaining high norepinephrine and dopamine levels to sustain your high-energy lifestyle. Then one day the demands and the lifestyle stop. The gas-pedal brain chemicals fall precipitously, leaving you feeling weak, purposeless, tired, and used up. Low norepinephrine levels by themselves can cause depression. If the holiday went badly, you may also suffer from low serotonin, caused by feelings of failure and low self-esteem.

People who suffer from such depressions often retreat into Satiation activities. Many withdraw from stimuli and watch a lot of television. They become chronically fatigued, directionless, and despairing. Some abuse alcohol or drugs. They have Satiation depression. As we will see, it is treated by raising serotonin while gradually increasing norepinephrine.

Others may try to maintain a hectic schedule artificially, refusing to let up for fear that they will fall into the despair of which they are vaguely aware. Many people drive themselves relentlessly until they become ill; this, of course, forces them to deal with both the illness and the underlying depression. This is Arousal depression. It is treated by lowering norepinephrine gradually, while increasing serotonin.

No matter what the situational cause—loss, workaholism, or long-term emotional stress—the first step in dealing with the condition is to determine whether you are experiencing a Satiation or an Arousal depression. Then you can take steps to alleviate your condition.

Finally, people with situational depression should take a look at their trigger situations, though this is less of a concern for them than for genetically and conditionally depressed people. Certain situations are going to remind you of the events that brought on your depression and therefore may reinforce the condition. Such triggers must be understood and dealt with effectively. By changing your brain chemistry and increasing your self-understanding, the programs described in Part Two of this book will help you create appropriate strategies for coping with such situations.

Before you can deal with your triggers, you need to understand how you cope with life in general. To accomplish this, we will look next at the two personality types, Satiation and Arousal, and the very distinct kinds of depression each type suffers.

Chapter 3

The Satiation
and Arousal
Personality Types

F or the vast majority of people, depression begins
with an internal and/or external conflict that remains unresolved for an extended period of time.
No matter what the original source of this conflict is, it eventually affects their decisions and every part of their life. The conflict itself becomes enlarged and takes center stage in the person's consciousness.
It feels like "the way life is," and the person believes she is powerless to
change the circumstances or her view of things in order to make herself happy. She begins to live with the most bitter of beliefs: "I must
live in an environment that does not support my existence and my
happiness—and I cannot change it." Whether in fact she has the power
to change her life is beside the point; she *believes* that she cannot

change the conditions. And this is enough to create the next stage of degeneration, which is hopelessness.

Hopelessness is overwhelmingly painful. Everyone has experienced it at various times; it is certainly a kind of hell. Hopelessness is a barred door that slams shut right in front of you. The pain is so terrible and so acute that it cannot be borne for very long. One of our adaptive responses to hopelessness is depression. Depression offers a reprieve from the intense pain of hopelessness. Don't get me wrong—depression is terrible, but hopelessness as an acute and ever-present conscious state is worse. Escape from hopelessness is essential, either through some sort of psychological disorder—depression is one example—or through overeating or some other method.

Depression, then, is a coping mechanism. It is true that for some depressed people hopelessness does resurface to drive them to engage in unwanted behaviors. And while depressed, all of us are still aware that life feels hopeless. But now the sense of hopelessness has been drained of some of its power by depression. Depression is a kind of sleep—a terrible dream perhaps, where the sun doesn't rise and the night offers no excitement. While depressed, we live in a numbed and barren world, where the life force has been drained from the past, present, and future. But looked at psychologically and physiologically, it is a condition that takes us out of an even more painful state and gives us time to review, adapt, and change.

All of these events change brain chemistry. In fact, the process that I have just described can establish a new baseline brain chemistry for a person, which in turn changes the way he perceives life. Debilitating events, such as the loss of a job or a loved one, can lower serotonin, and if these low serotonin levels are sustained long enough, they are perceived by the brain as normal. Once the brain recognizes the new chemical configuration—with its characteristically low serotonin levels—as the standard condition, it will sustain those levels. We may even become so familiar with the feelings arising from this new brain chemistry that they form the basis for our new identity. In effect, we may say to ourselves, "This is who I am. These feelings are normal for me." When low serotonin is maintained over time, we have the biochemical basis for chronic depression.

But this is only one type of baseline and only one type of depression. Another very common way in which the baseline can be altered is if a person finds herself in a stressful situation for a lengthy period of time. Take, for example, the person who is in a high-pressure job that does not give her a true sense of safety and satisfaction. Soon, she finds herself working hard to maintain her position in the company, which she feels is always threatened. These conditions raise norepinephrine and dopamine significantly and keep them elevated over time. Since these are adverse and unpleasant conditions, serotonin levels fall. Eventually, the person's baseline is changed so that high norepinephrine and low serotonin become the norm. At this point, she may have so much nervous tension and anxiety that she does not realize she's also depressed. She considers stress and tension normal from both a biochemical and a psychological perspective. She perceives herself as a person who's normally under a lot of pressure and tension. If she succeeds at meeting the challenges of her job, she gets certain psychological rewards—namely, greater status and more pay—which only serve to reinforce her existing beliefs, her behaviors, and her new baseline.

Before she entered this high-stress job, this person may have been happy-go-lucky and well equipped to enjoy a wide variety of experiences in life. But as her burdens at work have increased, her life has become more narrow. She may not see that there is any other way to live, which promotes an underlying feeling of hopelessness. Yet she avoids feeling such hopelessness and despair by maintaining her high-pressure schedule, keeping her stress and norepinephrine levels up. Eventually, she may have a heart attack or some other crisis that awakens her to her underlying depression. Until then, she is using stress and anxiety to medicate herself and thus avoid feeling her pain.

The Neurochemical and Psychological Reward System

Once our biochemical baseline has changed—once we feel that "this is me," even if this means that we are depressed—the brain resists further change. The new brain chemistry is now the basis for our identity, and we are rewarded biologically and often psychologically when we maintain that identity. One of the ways we are rewarded biologically is through the release of endorphins, those morphinelike substances that we mentioned in the last chapter. Endorphins provide temporary states of pleasure, relief from pain, and elevated feelings of well-being and satisfaction. They are *neuropeptides*, chains of amino acids that the brain releases to tell us that what we are doing feels good. All our experiences—everything from eating a meal, working, or engaging in sexual activity to experiencing moods, thoughts, memories, hunger, and satisfaction—either cause the release of endorphins or restrict their release, thus helping us discern whether an experience is pleasurable, rewarding, boring, uncomfortable, or harmful. This is one of the ways we decide what is pleasurable for us and what causes us pain. In the process, we develop routines, habits, and an identity.

As all of us know, not everything in our identities is healthful or gives us happiness. Yet the characteristics that do not particularly enhance our health are still supported because they are familiar and "normal" for us. An alcoholic is rewarded biochemically every time he drinks—serotonin levels rise for short periods, and endorphins are released—but maintaining this habit may well destroy him. Everyone who has overcome alcoholism or drug addiction knows that life under the spell of addiction is far worse than when one is free. Yet many of those who are addicted cannot imagine another life for themselves. Our sense of identity attempts to sustain itself through a biochemical reward system that includes the release of endorphins. To change, we have to confront parts of ourselves that are biochemically sustained, and this is partly why growth is resisted, at least initially.

Another biological way we maintain our baseline is through the release of neurotransmitters that discourage us from change. All of us are used to doing things in certain ways. Some of our behaviors are habitual. Acting in ways that are not familiar, normal, or habitual often causes insecurity and fear, and these feelings in turn elevate norepinephrine and dopamine. These chemicals take us out of a relaxed state and place us on alert. Biochemically and psychologically, we sense danger. Therefore, behaviors that are new and different are often associated with discomfort and even fear.

This entire cycle can be triggered by major as well as mundane changes, such as changing your hairstyle or the kinds of clothing you're used to wearing. For example, say you customarily dress for work in suits and fitted, formal clothing, but suddenly you change your style to include looser clothes that are more flowing and relaxed. You may have made this change because you perceive yourself as too stiff and bound up; you want to become more relaxed and more comfortable with your body, let's say. But the minute you put on these new clothes—no matter how good they make you feel—you become self-conscious and begin to worry about what other people will say. Your coworkers are used to seeing you in certain outfits. Will they accept the new you? What will they say behind your back? Will they criticize or make fun of you? Suddenly, dopamine and norepinephrine are skyrocketing. You are stressed; you perceive danger. Yet all you did was change the style of your clothing, and no one at work has even seen you, much less made a comment yet.

This is how brain chemistry works, however. It seeks to maintain what we take to be "normal" in even the most mundane and ordinary aspects of our lives. This is partly why we maintain behaviors over a long period of time, even when those behaviors do not make us feel good anymore.

Of course, there are also psychological rewards for maintaining what we perceive to be normal. Psychologically, we may be uncomfortable with certain changes because they violate long-held patterns, some of which were taught to us by our parents. Say your doctor tells you that your cholesterol level is too high and it has to come down right away. So you decide to throw away your mother's recipe for chicken-fried steak or sausage meatballs or sour cream sauce. Rather than feeling elated over your falling cholesterol level, you struggle with the guilt of betraying your mother. Rationally, you may know you're doing the right thing—even your mother would be happy that you're maintaining your health—but psychologically the change feels uncomfortable.

Usually, changing established behavior patterns is difficult because such change runs us up against both neurochemical and psychological boundaries. For example, let's say that you feel you must work very hard to prove your value to your coworkers and employer. After a time, you realize that you are exhausted and that your life is thoroughly out of balance. All you're doing is giving, giving, giving, and your efforts are not even appreciated. In fact, you sense you're being taken advantage of. Your first reaction is to get angry at yourself and those around you. Then you decide to change your behavior to bring your life more into balance. However, once you begin to change, a host of powerful feelings emerges to weaken your resolve. The first thing you realize is that you do not feel good about yourself when you're not driving yourself. The second feeling to emerge is fear: what if I'm perceived as someone who isn't carrying her fair share at work? I could lose my job.

The first feeling is a psychological disincentive against change, based on low self-esteem. In your own eyes you need to do more in order to feel worthy of your position at work. Chances are very good that this feeling comes from things you were taught as a child; these beliefs were probably not true then and are likely to be untrue today. Yet because they are strong beliefs, maintained by both psychological and biological rewards, they have always been difficult to change. Perhaps you have never allowed yourself to take a more balanced approach to your work, so you do not know what it would be like to give your job a different priority in your life. Yet your belief system tells you that you *do* know what it would be like if your work occupied less than, say, 80 percent of your life. Your belief system tells you that you would be out of a job and that life would be terrible. This, of course, has prevented you from changing.

The second feeling is largely a neurochemical disincentive to change: new behaviors bring on unfamiliar experiences, which trigger the release of norepinephrine and a consequent increase in anxiety, tension, and fear. These psychological and neurochemical responses to change work in concert; we have separated them here just to make them really clear. In fact, the psychological sense of low self-esteem, which is associated with low serotonin, can trigger feelings of distress and anxiety, which in turn produce higher levels of norepinephrine. Generally speaking, all change—no matter how high our confidence may be—triggers an increase in norepinephrine and dopamine, with related increases in stress, anxiety, and fear.

Change and the Creation of a New Baseline

Neurochemical and psychological rewards and resistances exist throughout our lives and serve to sustain what we regard as our normal identity. Anything that you do that feels out of the ordinary causes you some psychological and neurochemical discomfort, as you try to determine whether this change is good or bad for you and whether or not it should be maintained.

This raises an interesting challenge for most of us: one of the ways in which we resist change is by visualizing that the new condition will be worse than the existing one. For depressed people, it's often difficult to realize that depression isn't normal and that by changing their behaviors, they will not become an even smaller or weaker version of themselves. The underlying sense of hopelessness that goes with the condition prevents people from seeing that by changing their behavior, they can become happier, healthier, and far more effective at everything they do. Thus, in order to change, we must first confront our dark or negative beliefs about the future. Such images, of course, are projections of our own fears. They must be confronted and overcome if we are to escape the dark world of depression.

But it isn't just our projections that we must confront. Change forces us to grapple with the feelings that arise from our altered brain chemistry. Let's go back to my example of the hardworking person who has neglected her own needs and suddenly decides to start enjoying life a little more. The feelings of fear and insecurity that naturally arise from such a change must be endured if they are to be overcome. The person must discover that working fewer hours and developing outside interests do not bring on the loss of her job. On the contrary, enjoying life may well help her to do a better job and will certainly make her an easier person to work with. But before such discoveries can be made, she must be willing to tolerate some discomfort while she explores a new reality.

Meanwhile, what is happening biochemically? Let's say that our hardworking person starts to enjoy music, or theater, or a new sport, or greater intimacy with friends and even herself. All of these are serotonin boosters. They will also be calming, which means they will lower norepinephrine. In effect, she is balancing out her workaholic pattern by incorporating more calming and nurturing activities. If such behaviors are maintained, a new baseline will be established with higher serotonin and lower norepinephrine, meaning the person will experience greater confidence, a stronger sense of well-being, and lower stress.

Any break with customary ways of being causes the release of powerful emotions and with them dramatic changes in brain chemistry. Midlife crises, divorce, and changing careers all alter brain chemistry and, over time, establish a new baseline that can cause changes in personality. If the person truly confronts those characteristics within him that have helped to give rise to the crisis, he has a chance of changing his baseline for the better and emerging as a healthier, more balanced, and stronger individual. Consistency changes the baseline. Whatever you think, believe, and do consistently will establish a new brain chemistry, and this will give rise to certain feelings that eventually you will regard as normal.

Once you are willing to change, you are ready to ask such fundamental questions as "What do I need to change to reestablish balance in my life?" and "How can I make such changes?" To answer these questions, we must first understand the kinds of imbalances we suffer from. Or to put it another way, we must understand whether we are a Satiation or an Arousal type.

Your Response to Conflict

Depression has its seeds in an internal conflict and our response to that conflict. Broadly speaking, there are two primary responses to conflict: fight or flight. Either we confront the conflict and its causes directly, or we run. Some will say that a third option is simply to endure the conflict, but when we examine endurance a little more closely we recognize that it is either a strategy for fighting—one endures but remains vigilant until that moment when he can advance and change the conditions—or a way to flee or retreat. But if endurance represents an endless retreat, it eventually will lead to depression because no positive action has been taken to change the circumstances. Endurance is an important strategy, but the underlying attitude determines the effect that endurance has on us: are we enduring in order to fight tomorrow, or are we enduring in order to avoid the challenges that confront us?

Whether we fight or flee is determined to a great extent by our biochemical makeup. These characteristics also form behavior patterns that we recognize as part of our normal identity. All of us have some degree of imbalance in our natures that causes us to lean more toward passivity or aggression. A few of us are balanced—that is, we can be passive at times and aggressive at others. But most of us tend to lean one way or the other; usually we respond to conflict with some form of passivity or with some form of aggression, whether it is intellectual, emotional, or physical.

Passivity and aggression are symptoms of larger psychological and biochemical profiles that each of us fit into, profiles I call Satiation and Arousal. The vast majority of us—even those who are not depressed—are either a Satiation-type personality or an Arousal type. Each type of personality, however, is susceptible to a specific type of depression, which I refer to as a Satiation depression or an Arousal depression. In order to know which program to adopt to manage and overcome your depression, you first need to know which of the two personality types—Satiation or Arousal—is yours.

As you read the descriptions of these types, please keep in mind that they are slightly exaggerated one-sided representations of each personality. Most of us are combinations of the Satiation and Arousal types; our basic nature simply leans a bit more toward one or the other. Ideally, we should be balanced between the two, since both have characteristics that make personal fulfillment and success possible. But very few of us were born with such a balance. We are genetically programmed with either more Satiation or more Arousal traits, and this allows us to categorize ourselves as one or the other.

The Satiation Personality: Let's Smell the Roses

The Satiation personality is characterized by the ongoing effort to boost serotonin to promote relaxation, concentration, and feelings of safety, security, and well-being. Satiation personalities are attracted to relaxed environments, places that have a calm atmosphere, such as a library, a cozy restaurant, one's bedroom, or one's living room when the television is off. Many love to read and listen to calming music.

Satiation personalities are driven to achieve intimacy with themselves and others. They are commonly referred to as "type B" personalities (the opposite of the goal-oriented, driven "type A"); they tend to focus on relationships more than on accomplishments. They prefer environments and activities that allow people to get to know each other. Even when they are engaged in some active sport or recreational activity, they prefer playing with only one or two other people, because this allows for greater emotional intimacy. Satiation types love lengthy, intimate, intellectual conversations; they do not enjoy competitive or passionate debates. When faced with conflict, they tend to respond with gentleness and passivity. They like to calm turbulent waters, and they see themselves as peacemakers.

In general, Satiation types emphasize the importance of the past and present, rather than the future.

Satiation types abhor stress; many will do everything possible to avoid it. This gets them into trouble in numerous ways. Some duck responsibility for situations that may be stressful but must be confronted. Others manipulate events or people in order to escape demanding situations.

If their jobs force them to confront stress, they will adapt and may become workaholics, but they will never be fully satisfied with their workaholism; in other words, they will always harbor an internal conflict over the sacrifices they have made for the job. When Satiation types are driven to workaholism, it is usually to compensate for their depression. They want to be appreciated for what they do but do not want to call attention to themselves. Very often, these characteristics make the Satiation person wonder if he isn't being taken advantage of or overlooked. Such feelings cause great internal conflict and sometimes bitterness.

Satiation types enjoy exercises that promote relaxation, such as walking, swimming, bicycle riding, and low-impact aerobics. If they engage in a vigorous sport, it will usually be aerobic and introverting or meditative, such as jogging or cross-country skiing. In general, Satiation types prefer noncompetitive sports; when they play a competitive game, they focus more on themselves than on conquering their opponent. They are more likely to play the "inner game": they concentrate on skill development, self-improvement, and maintaining emotional equilibrium. Golf is a favorite game among Satiation types.

Because they are trying to relax, Satiation personalities are vulnerable to addictions that anesthetize the mind and body. The most common of these are television watching, excessive sugar consumption, alcohol abuse, and the use of marijuana. They are also prone to perfectionism, wanting everything to be in its proper place. Satiation types can rigidly adhere to routines and their own definitions of order. Having things in their place and holding to specific habits gives them a sense of safety and security, while any disruption to their habits and routines can be very upsetting. All of these characteristics can cause them to resist change stubbornly.

As the name implies, Satiation types eat to experience satiety; their preferred food by far is carbohydrates, which promote the production of serotonin. Their diets are dominated by pasta, flour products (such as bread, muffins, rolls, and pastries), and sugar. They like protein foods, such as red meat, chicken, and eggs, but these foods are in the minority. They love soft dairy products, such as ice cream, soft cheeses, and sauces. They especially like chocolate, and they often snack until late at night. Because alcohol is a powerful serotonin booster, Satiation personalities may be strongly attracted to beer and wine (many are connoisseurs of wine and food). On the other hand, they usually avoid hard liquors, which are too powerful for the passive and introverted Satiation personality.

Like their Arousal personality counterparts, Satiation types drink coffee and other caffeinated beverages to increase neurotransmission and promote gas-pedal chemicals in the brain. Many Satiation types use coffee and other caffeinated beverages as a drug to push themselves into confronting the workday. They'd rather be walking in the park, talking with a friend, or doing some hobby that they particularly enjoy. The work world is far too demanding and stressful for their tastes. They enter it out of necessity. Coffee, with its powerful effect on brain chemistry, allows them to keep up with their Arousal brethren.

Research has shown that coffee improves alertness, mental acuity, and concentration. It significantly enhances the brain's problem-solving abilities. It also elevates mood, boosts confidence, and makes people more optimistic, at least temporarily. Caffeine has an anti-depressant effect; for some people, it even produces euphoria. These effects occur for virtually all people, no matter whether they are daily caffeine consumers or only drink the stuff occasionally. Coffee also has negative side effects. Like other drugs that promote the production of gas-pedal chemicals, coffee eventually creates its opposite effect, caus-ing anxiety, physical tension, and, for many, mild but palpable fear.

Because coffee causes so much anxiety, some Satiation types avoid it entirely and choose black tea, which has between one-third and one-fourth the caffeine content of coffee (depending on how the tea and coffee are brewed).

Satiation types quickly become uncomfortable, tense, and threat-ened when situations become too arousing. They seek ways to escape such situations and return to their safe havens and routines. In general, Satiation personalities prefer boredom to excitement and mild depres-sion to anxiety. Any workday that is highly stimulating, exciting, or de-manding must be dealt with by withdrawing to the safety of home, quiet, and relaxation. As much as possible, Satiation types avoid foods and activities that increase norepinephrine and dopamine.

The Type of Depression Satiation Types Suffer

The danger facing Satiation types is that they can become too imbalanced on the Satiation side and thus suffer from what I call "downer depression," characterized by withdrawal, introversion, low energy, confusion, and fear of any sort of challenge or stressful event.

Satiation types become highly adept at recognizing in advance those kinds of situations that they believe will be stressful or demand-ing. As they get older, they tend to become more reclusive and cut off from others. In the same way, because they tolerate mild depression so well, they can easily fall into severe depression before they realize it.

Once Satiation-type individuals become depressed, they are typi-cally paralyzed by it. Since they avoid excitement, they unwittingly de-prive themselves of any situation that would boost norepinephrine and thereby restore a sense of personal power and lift their spirits. In a more balanced person who is used to enjoying both Satiation and Arousal activities, stimulating events would provide a reward, but for the Satiation type, such activities are anxiety producing and therefore avoided.

It's important to remember that if you are a Satiation personality and are currently depressed, you will still be a Satiation personality after you have overcome your depression. Being a Satiation or an Arousal type does not mean that you have a disorder. Both types are implicitly healthy; they are just vulnerable to different types of depression.

The Arousal Personality: Some Like It Hot

Arousal personalities choose foods and activities that promote production of norepinephrine and dopamine, the two gas-pedal neurotransmitters that create feelings of arousal, increased energy, alertness, assertiveness, and aggression. Arousal types are those who usually respond to conflict by confronting the situation and trying to control the events.

Arousal types enjoy all activities that provide excitement, increased energy, and stimulation. Norepinephrine and dopamine increase heart rate, respiration, and metabolism. Arousal types therefore always seem to be in motion. They like to speed up events and move quickly toward the realization of their goals. Arousal personalities are focused primarily on the future and to a lesser extent on the present. They care little about the past, except in terms of how it might affect the future or teach them how to achieve their desires. Arousal personalities are goal-oriented and are prone to becoming workaholics.

Arousal types are rewarded biochemically and psychologically by activity, stress, excitement, and success. They love to work hard, play hard, and party hard. They can be overtly ambitious. Many have no compunction about promoting themselves. They move toward their goals with directness and courage, though they can also be Machiavellian when it comes to office politics. They are risk takers and enjoy all kinds of daredevil activities, such as carnival rides and fast cars. In business and elsewhere in life, they tend to be gamblers.

Arousal types are not much attracted to intimacy or activities that promote intimacy. Rather than long conversations by the fire, Arousal personalities prefer an evening of dancing or a concert (for many, a rock concert). They like group activities in which three or more people participate. Consequently, Arousal types often have many friends and acquaintances but few if any intimate partners.

They are attracted to all sports and activities that promote norepinephrine and dopamine, such as competitive sports (they play to win), downhill skiing, bicycle riding (on hills), mountain climbing, and white-water rafting.

Arousal types can become addicted to the control and manipulation of events and people, and to cocaine (a norepinephrine and dopamine booster), gambling, sexual activity, and alcohol. Often Arousal types combine an arousing activity, such as gambling, with alcohol. The relaxation provided by the alcohol allows them to indulge even more in the stress of gambling.

Many Arousal personalities come from abusive families in which the child perceived an ongoing threat from his parents. That fear created a baseline in which norepinephrine and dopamine remained elevated. Children who are Arousal types are often misdiagnosed as having a learning disability or attention deficit disorders because they are unable to sit still for very long. These children may be inherently as intelligent as any child in the school, yet as long as their baselines are composed of extremely elevated norepinephrine and dopamine, they will have trouble sitting still.

On the other hand, Arousal types have great curiosity—they love the stimulation of new and exciting subjects or experiences—and are attracted to all kinds of information. This characteristic may make some of them dilettantes.

The diets of people with Arousal personalities consist of lots of protein-rich foods, which boost dopamine and norepinephrine levels. Steaks, hamburgers, hot dogs, sausages, eggs, and hard cheeses are all foods that promote the production of norepinephrine and dopamine.

As for entertainment, Arousal types like arousing music. They prefer Beethoven and Tchaikovsky to Bach and Chopin, New Orleans jazz and rock to folk and country. When they go on vacation, Arousal types go for the excitement, the activity, and the thrill of exotic locations.

Arousal types prefer anxiety to boredom. They fear depression, which causes many to run away from their feelings. Ironically, running from their feelings can lead to inner conflict and eventually to depression.

The Type of Depression Suffered by the Arousal Personality

Arousal personalities fall into the type of depression I call anxious depression, meaning that they are more aware of their anxiety than their depression. Depression is terrifying to the Arousal personality because it implies defeat. The Arousal person is constantly pushing toward his goals. Meanwhile, the other side of his nature—namely, the part of him that experiences emotions, needs love, and wants to give love—is calling out to him for attention. The psyche is always seeking balance between the Arousal and Satiation sides of our being. Unfortunately, the speed at which many Arousal people are moving prevents any real understanding of their Satiation needs. In effect, the Arousal side is repressing the Satiation side. But unlike the Satiation person, the Arousal person medicates herself by using stress to keep from feeling her underlying psychological pain.

This is very easy to accomplish for the Arousal personality, because she maintains a high-anxiety life. The immediate and acute condition she feels is anxiety, but beneath the anxiety is depression, brought on by the denial of her needs for peace, nurturance, and love.

In Summary

I have provided a chart that summarizes the characteristics and preferences of these two personality types. The goal for all of us is to become more balanced so that we can embrace both Satiation and Arousal activities. Only in this way can we enjoy a wide variety of experiences and have a fulfilling life.

Characteristics of the Two Personality Types

Satiation   Arousal

PERSONALITY TRAITS

Satiation	Arousal
• Is relationship-oriented	• Is a type A personality
• Is family-centered	• Is goal-oriented and highly ambitious
• Has moderate to low ambition	• Prefers many friends, new acquaintances, and new and exciting social situations in which he or she can meet new people
• Avoids conflict, represses anger, avoids expressing feelings that may cause antagonism	
• Is a type B	• Engages in activities that promote production of gas-pedal neurotransmitters, dopamine and norepinephrine
• Is vulnerable to downer depression	• Has little difficulty letting go of old relationships and getting on with life
• Prefers social situations that include one or two people as opposed to groups of three or more	• Enjoys changes in routine and often seeks change
• Prefers having close friends who are maintained over long periods as opposed to forming new and exciting relationships	• May have difficulty with intimacy and close relationships
	• May have difficulty looking inside self for answers to life questions
• Engages in activities that promote production of serotonin	• Prefers to change environment rather than change self
• Is very attached to daily routine	• Tends to emphasize career over family, though this may be unconscious and he or she may deny this strongly
	• Finds conflict stimulating, exciting, and arousing and therefore may seek it out
	• Will express anger, especially if dopamine levels are low
	• Seeks challenging or stressful situations, crisis, and difficult tasks, though this may be unconscious
	• Is prone to workaholism
	• Bases self-esteem on the achievement of goals and ambitions, thus raising the stakes of any undertaking to disproportionately high levels; goals and ambitions often eclipse other priorities in life

Characteristics of the Two Personality Types (continued)
Satiation   Arousal

TYPES OF WORK PREFERRED

Satiation

- Office work, preferably done alone or in small groups
- Work that requires low physical demands
- Jobs that do not involve high stress (unless stress is internally created as a drive for success)
- Regular working hours, with weekends, holidays, and birthday off (unless internal drives cause workaholism)
- Computer technician
- Librarian
- Homemaker
- Teacher, preferably of kindergarten and lower grades or college (Most college professors are Satiation types.)
- Research scientist
- Pediatrician, family doctor, internist, and general practitioner (as opposed to emergency room physician or surgeon)

Arousal

- Jobs that take place outdoors
- Jobs requiring physical activity and much change
- High-stress positions, even those that are relatively low on the ladder
- Police officer
- Rescue worker
- Politician
- Journalist
- Scientist with interest in public speaking or highly political positions
- Social activist
- Emergency room doctor, surgeon
- Consultant

FOODS PREFERRED

Satiation

- Sugar
- Sweet carbohydrate-rich foods, such as croissants, muffins, cakes, doughnuts
- Soft candy
- Chocolate
- Peanut butter and other nut butters
- Fruit
- Sweet dairy foods, such as ice cream, milk shakes, frozen yogurt
- Soft dairy foods, such as milk and soft cheeses like Brie and Camembert
- Pasta
- Soft grains, such as boiled rice, wheat, and barley

Arousal

- Protein-rich foods, such as red meat, hard cheeses, eggs, poultry
- Coffee
- Caffeinated soft drinks, such as colas
- Spicy foods
- Exotic foods
- Typical breakfast: eggs and meat; quick protein drink; coffee
- Typical lunch: hamburger; sub sandwich; French fries; caffeinated soft drinks
- Typical dinner: meat; potatoes; dessert; alcohol; coffee

Satiation	Arousal

FOODS PREFERRED (continued)

- Beer

- Wine

- Typical breakfast: toast; English muffin; cereal; tea

- Typical lunch: salad; chicken sandwich

- Typical dinner: pasta; fish; chicken

TYPES OF EXERCISE PREFERRED

Satiation	Arousal
• Walking	• Vigorous exercise
• Stretching	• Running
• Swimming	• Highly arousing, aerobic, and high-risk sports: downhill skiing, water skiing, basketball, racquetball, skateboarding, bicycling, ice hockey, hang gliding
• Low-impact aerobics	
• Long-distance running	
	• Doing aerobics to music

TYPES OF ENTERTAINMENT PREFERRED

Satiation	Arousal
• Films: love stories, romantic dramas, comedies, foreign films, and light feel-good movies	• Dancing
	• Improvisational theater
• Dinners out in intimate settings	• Parties
• Long talks	• Karaoke
• Museums	• Rock concerts
• Symphony concerts	• Sporting events, especially football and basketball games, ice hockey, and boxing matches
• Theater: intellectual dramas and feel-good musicals	
• Music preferences: folk, light rock, meditative classical music	

RECREATIONAL OR PRESCRIPTION DRUGS THEY ARE MOST LIKELY TO TAKE

Satiation	Arousal
• Marijuana	• Cocaine
• Barbiturates	• Amphetamines (such as speed)
• Anti-depressants, such as Prozac	• Ritalin
• Anti-anxiety drugs, such as Valium, Xanax, others	• Over-the-counter diet pills

Characteristics of the Two Personality Types (continued)
Satiation   Arousal

RECREATIONAL OR PRESCRIPTION DRUGS
THEY ARE MOST LIKELY TO TAKE (continued)

Satiation	Arousal
• Vacations that are low on activity, high on relaxation	• Vacations in big cities (especially New York, New Orleans, and San Francisco)
• Time with family at a private beach or in a relaxed country setting	• Downhill skiing
• Places where time slows down	• Waterskiing
	• Big family reunions
	• Group tours to exotic locations around the world
	• African safaris
	• Hunting

BEST FORMS FOR ACHIEVING INSIGHT

Satiation	Arousal
• One-on-one counseling	• Active listening
• Counseling in small groups of two or three	• Large group workshops
• Talking-based, rather than activity-based	• Recreational or weekend activity retreats
• Religion and spiritual practices: low arousal, highly meditative, relaxing, internal	
• Self-help books and tapes	

Finding Your Neurochemical Personality Type

Knowing whether you are a Satiation or an Arousal personality type will help you determine which of the programs in Part Two of this book is appropriate for you.

You have probably already recognized yourself in the descriptions of either the Satiation or the Arousal personality, but in order to confirm your suspicion, I have provided the following questionnaire.

Please answer "yes" or "no" to all twenty-four questions. If you are uncertain about the answer to any question, use "yes" if you feel a "yes" answer is generally true and "no" if the answer is generally "no."

➤ Satiation Versus Arousal Questionnaire

1. Do you choose activities that require active participation?
2. Do you find yourself reacting more strongly to situations when you are stressed or depressed?
3. Are you comfortable socializing with large groups of people?
4. Have you felt that you were not promoted at your job because of a particular behavior, incident, or action you engaged in?
5. Do you enjoy watching movies in which violence plays a part?
6. Do you enjoy gambling?
7. Do you frequently buy lottery tickets or bet on sporting events?
8. Do you tend to drink alcohol or use drugs (including caffeine and nicotine) in social settings?
9. Do you get pleasure or feel good after using drugs that increase your energy level (including nicotine and caffeine)?
10. Do you feel good when you engage in risk-oriented activities (such as speeding, mountain climbing, hang gliding, racing)?
11. When you feel stressed, do activities that require lots of energy relax you?
12. Do you prefer to participate in groups (including religious groups) with strong beliefs and a high level of emotional involvement?
13. Do you like being involved in a small, close-knit group, where you feel a sense of intimacy and warmth?
14. Do you usually continue to eat even after you are full or feel you have had enough?

y 15. Do you tend to eat when you are depressed, anxious, or angry?

y 16. Do you use alcohol or drugs to relax?

y 17. Do you use quieting activities to decrease your anxiety?

y 18. Do you try to find ways to avoid conflict?

n 19. On average, do you watch more than fifteen hours of television a week?

n 20. Do you go to the movies or watch movies on TV at least twice weekly?

n 21. Do you rent videotapes at least once a week?

y 22. When depressed, do you participate in quieting activities to increase your energy?

y 23. Are you a member of or do you participate in groups (including religious groups) that have strict ethics, rules, or codes of behavior?

y 24. Do you spend much of your free time alone?

Scoring

1. Add your "yes" answers for 1–12 and put the total here:

   5 _____

2. Add your "yes" answers for 13–24 and put the total here:

   9 _____

If you had more "yes" answers to questions 1–12, you are an Arousal personality.

If you had more "yes" answers to 13–24, you are a Satiation personality.

If the number of "yes" answers equals the number of "no" answers, review the characteristics of each personality type and choose the one you feel more closely describes you.

I am a/an _____ _____ personality.

Satiation

In this chapter, I have touched on the fact that out of the Satiation and Arousal personalities come very specific types of depressions, each a reflection of an underlying brain-chemistry imbalance. Both types of depression arise out of the need to control events—one through passivity and retreat, the other through aggression and direct intervention—in order to feel safe. And both emerge from specific underlying beliefs and conflicts that change brain chemistry and give rise to depression.

Let's turn now to the conflicts and beliefs related to the Satiation and Arousal personalities and look more closely at the kinds of depression these characteristics create.

Chapter 4

The Satiation-
Depressed
Personality

Joe was raised by parents who were continually fighting and threatening each other with divorce. For as long as he can remember, Joe struggled to decide with whom he would live if his parents separated. Sometimes he would fantasize about appearing in divorce court and telling the judge which of his parents was right or wrong in a particular argument. This image came from television shows he had seen in which parents fought over the custody of their children, only to have the children themselves decide with whom they would live. In Joe's fantasy, the judge always accepted Joe's analysis of the situation and settled the dispute as Joe would have liked. Despite the relief his fantasy offered, his parents' fighting got Joe down. When they finally divorced—Joe was twelve at the time—he retreated into fantasy novels, his schoolwork, and the world of his imagination. Looking back, Joe says that he was clearly depressed by the time he reached his teenage years. It was not the kind of overt depression that calls attention to itself, he told me many years later. It was more withdrawn, moody, and hurt. This condition lingered throughout his adolescence.

Joe didn't date for very long before he was married at the age of twenty. He was hoping for the fantasy relationship that he had always pictured in his mind, but the marriage couldn't live up to that image, and the two divorced after four years together. They had no children.

Joe was depressed throughout his marriage. He had little energy, felt confused much of the time, and was unable to communicate effectively with his wife. He spent a lot of his free time watching television. I had Joe complete my Mood Optimization Survey (found in the back of this book) and found him to be low in both serotonin and norepinephrine. He suffered from what I call conditioned Satiation depression, meaning that he was a Satiation personality whose depression emerged from patterns acquired in childhood. His response to these conditions—withdrawal, confusion, low energy, and isolation—were all consistent with the Satiation type and the kind of "downer depression" that results from low serotonin and low norepinephrine.

Well after his divorce, Joe speculated that perhaps he had married young in order to have someone with whom he could work out his childhood issues. Yet some psychological and biochemical barrier prevented him from confronting the problems of his marriage and those of his childhood. This barrier consisted of his refusal to enter situations that were arousing and that demanded he examine the conditioning and pain of his past. When faced with marital problems, Joe repeated the pattern he had established as a child: he retreated from the pain through avoidance, fantasy, and isolation. He ate lots of sweets and other junk foods and did not exercise. In this way, Joe maintained his existing baseline brain chemistry, which was centered entirely around short-term serotonin-boosting foods and activities, while avoiding arousing activities that would increase norepinephrine.

Not surprisingly, these very strategies left him feeling powerless, hopeless, and depressed. What other effect could they have? If Joe had confronted his wife with their problems, he would have had to say something like "It makes me feel bad when you do such-and-such." His wife may have retorted, "Why does that make you feel bad?" With some self-examination, he probably would have said something like "Well, I don't like it when you do it. But it also reminds me of when I was a little kid and my mother used to do that and my father got angry, and then they started fighting and I felt terrible. I just wanted them to be quiet and be nice to each other." His wife might have replied, "I am not your mother and I don't like it when you sit around so much of the time watching television and spacing out. Why do you do that? Why don't we talk or go out more and do things?" At this point, Joe might have been forced to face his dilemma. He might have had to say, "I get upset inside whenever I talk about my feelings. Sometimes, I get stressed when we go out, too. I really don't want to do very much. I feel like sitting around a lot, so I watch television or eat to distract me from what I'm feeling." When confronted by the truth of Joe's inner condition, his wife could have said, "Well, we have to find out why you lack motivation and feel nervous and stressed out whenever you talk about your feelings. Maybe we need help."

This could have been the beginning of Joe's journey to health. The more the two explored the dynamics between them, the greater the likelihood that both Joe and his wife would have been drawn deeper into their own individual and personal issues. In the process, Joe would have been led directly into his old pain, which would have been disturbing and arousing but would also have opened up the possibility of understanding himself more deeply and being able to change old patterns that were no longer healthy for him, especially in his marriage. As he became more aroused by his confrontation with himself and his new insights, norepinephrine and dopamine would have increased, which in time would have changed Joe's baseline brain chemistry, making him more assertive and confident.

When I asked Joe how he felt about his role in his marriage and divorce, he used words like "awful," "ashamed," "powerless," and "failure." Joe found it painful just looking back on the past. Yet he had no plan for changing the future, at least not one that he could follow for very long. This is typical of Satiation-depressed people. They are haunted by the past, yet they have no strategy for making the future any different. Thus, they feel isolated and powerless in the present. As long as he refused to confront his old pain, Joe could not grow beyond the childhood belief that he was powerless to create a future that differed from his past. This, of course, only contributed to his feelings of hopelessness and depression.

One of the reasons he could not confront his old pain was that he was extremely uncomfortable with any increase in norepinephrine, which he experienced as intolerable anxiety and fear. As a child, arousing situations were exploding all the time. Confrontation was frightening to Joe; it drove him back into his shell. On some level, Joe was always wishing that his childhood had been different, that he had been raised by loving and caring parents. He had to grieve the loss of that dream and accept that he would never have the happy childhood for which he longed. But even more, he would have to change his way of dealing with the present; this meant that he would have to establish a more balanced brain chemistry, which would give him a sense of power, control, and assertiveness. In other words, gradually but steadily, he would have to increase both serotonin and norepinephrine.

The details of Joe's life are unique, just as the details of yours and mine are. Yet Joe has many similarities with all Satiation personality types who fall into depression. Joe's personality had become too one-sided. He engaged too often in activities that made him feel safe and protected him from feelings of anxiety, frustration, anger, and rage. In the process, he became too withdrawn and introverted. In terms of our brain-chemistry model, Joe became disproportionately engaged in short-term serotonin-boosting activities, while avoiding activities that would maintain normal levels of norepinephrine. He cut off a whole part of himself—and of life itself—a part of himself that was essential to the experience of fulfillment and satisfaction. In short, he prevented himself from becoming whole.

Joe's experience serves as an object lesson for us all. The body, mind, and spirit demand balance and wholeness. From a brain-chemistry standpoint, this means that we need to balance our Satiation and Arousal sides—that is, our serotonin and norepinephrine levels. It is true that very few of us will ever achieve perfect balance between the two. In fact, most of us will remain either a Satiation type or an Arousal type, but we must still be able to enjoy the kinds of behaviors that are the opposite of our type. For the Satiation personality, this means being able to engage in the world and deal effectively with arousing situations. For the Arousal type, it means being able to rest and to experience intimacy and love, putting aside one's ambitions, goals, and work agenda.

All of us—whether we are Satiation or Arousal types—must be willing to experience our underlying feelings if we are to be healthy. The opposite tactic—the mammoth effort of denying our inner conflicts and emotions and of establishing behavioral patterns that help us avoid self-awareness—leads to depression.

Satiation Depression: Low Neurochemistry and Low Energy

In general, the brain chemistry of a Satiation-depressed personality is low in serotonin and low in norepinephrine and dopamine. When serotonin and norepinephrine fall below a certain threshold, which is unique to each individual, Satiation depression sets in. This brain-chemical configuration creates the kind of depression characterized by lethargy, confusion, withdrawal, and an inability to concentrate. The person becomes excessively passive and too inwardly focused. It's as if her life force were turning inward, imploding. There is a complete lack of assertiveness, determination, and aggression. The rate of neurotransmission, or the speed with which she thinks, will also be slower, thanks to the low norepinephrine and dopamine. Consequently, she's a bit slow to respond to stimuli from the environment. Insufficient serotonin alone will lower her self-esteem, confidence, and sense of well-being. When low serotonin is combined with low norepinephrine, the decrease in confidence is even more pronounced. Such a person tends to doubt his native intelligence because he feels just a step or two slower than others. He can also be frustrated by the realization that he doesn't react well or rapidly to changing situations and unexpected events. Often he fails to say or do things that later he wishes he had said or done. This, of course, causes him to place all the more emphasis on the past. This is also a distinguishing characteristic of Satiation-depressed people: they overemphasize the past and feel frustrated and shamed by events that often they had little or no control over.

The lower norepinephrine and dopamine levels are, the less assertive and energetic the person will be. If norepinephrine and dopamine are very low, the person can become exceedingly introverted and suffer from a kind of vegetative, or downer, depression. She'll feel as if there just isn't enough fuel in her tank to meet life's demands. In time, such people become more and more withdrawn and negative.

Typically, Satiation-depressed people try to avoid arousing situations that would raise norepinephrine and dopamine levels. As this behavior becomes more habitual, the person avoids all activities that excite, arouse, and give rise to the unexpected, thus excluding all those activities and foods that raise norepinephrine and dopamine. As their baseline norepinephrine levels fall even further, their ability to tolerate excitement and arousal drops as well. This cycle leads inevitably to depression.

For the Satiation personality, depression begins with an insidious belief that he or she can establish harmony, safety, and peace by controlling the environment through *behaviors designed to avoid conflict and arousing situations*. The top two priorities for Satiation types are

(1) to achieve peace within their relationships and (2) to gain the respect of their peers. In the depressed person, neither of these can be fully realized because of the misperceptions created by their imbalanced brain chemistry. Let's look at the most common misperceptions that shape the Satiation-depressed person's life.

Control and the Pursuit of Safety

Satiation-depressed people are secretly terrified of change and do everything in their power to establish security and stability in their worlds. This often leads them to believe that they can somehow control their environments sufficiently to avoid arousing situations. They use many different strategies for controlling situations and people, all of which are unique to this personality type.

One of the ways they try to create such security is by clinging tenaciously to their routines. They regard the status quo as safe, even when it is filled with all kinds of difficult conditions. As I suggested earlier, to them the hell that is known is far better than the one that's unknown.

In order to reinforce the status quo, many Satiation-depressed people schedule themselves tightly. They fill up their days with activities they know to be safe. They make lists of what they must do each day and adhere to these lists as if they were sacred. Anyone who causes them to violate their routines or not fulfill their list of "things to do today" is severely disliked and usually subjected to their smoldering but unspoken hostility.

Their most common response to demands or conflict from their environment is simply to avoid it. Procrastination is a common tool for avoiding any situation that they perceive to be too demanding.

Achieving peace and stability in relationships is terribly important to all Satiation types and particularly to the Satiation person who is chronically depressed. This provides him with the love he is seeking as well as the security that enhances serotonin production and maintains his baseline. The negative emotions of others, such as anger, moodiness, or irritability—all of which, ironically, are commonly exhibited by Satiation-depressed people—create insecurity and therefore boost norepinephrine and dopamine in Satiation types. This, of course, is intolerable for the Satiation-depressed person.

One of the most common ways for Satiation-depressed people to control their environment and others is by becoming a people pleaser. Generally, they do this by being gentle and nonconfrontational, avoiding conflict at all cost. Some become overly positive, never expressing their own needs or desires. They especially avoid anger—either their own or that of others—because anger is unpredictable and arousing; in other words, it boosts norepinephrine. Their people pleasing is intended to create security. The thinking goes something like this: "If everyone loves me, I'll never have to deal with their anger, hostility, or criticism. Having everyone like me gives me positive feedback from others and makes the world safe for me. Being nice to people creates safety. Therefore, it works."

Another common approach for Satiation personalities—especially when they are depressed—is to become overly negative and cynical about people, situations, and the future. This keeps them from having to commit their energy, creativity, and hope to any situation or relationship. It is another way of protecting themselves and controlling their environment. The thinking goes something like this: "People can't be counted on. They always betray me. Therefore, I must never commit myself, my hopes, or my energy to any person or situation."

Being overly positive or overly negative is, in fact, a kind of withdrawal of one's true self from life. It's an entirely one-sided approach to life, based on the fundamental misperception that such a one-sided approach can create safety. As every adult knows, goodness and weakness exist in everyone; similarly, every situation—no matter how good or bad—contains difficulties and opportunities. Moreover, each of us helps to create—by our own efforts, behaviors, and attitudes—the outcome and the quality of every situation we find ourselves in. Both a discriminating eye and a positive outlook are essential to the success of any endeavor. When we are either overly amenable or overly negative, one of these essential ingredients is missing.

Withdrawal of one kind or another is perhaps the most common strategy among Satiation-depressed people. Usually this withdrawal consists simply of avoiding relationships, challenges, and adventures altogether. Satiation-depressed people pull back from social situations and become introverted. This will decrease norepinephrine and dopamine, but the powerlessness that results from the reduction of these neurotransmitters also causes a diminished sense of security. This creates a downward spiral, in which these people suffer an ever-increasing sense of fear, insecurity, and danger, feelings that cause many to keep withdrawing until they become shut-ins and recluses.

Withdrawal can also be accomplished through addiction to a Satiation behavior, such as television watching; consumption of sugar, other refined carbohydrates, and chocolate; or the use of alcohol and drugs, especially marijuana. Another form of withdrawal is to become a hypochondriac. Sickness becomes a means of escaping full participation in—and responsibility for—any socially demanding task. Hypochondria is often coupled with feelings of self-pity.

In the end, the Satiation-depressed person feels he is driven to withdrawal by the overwhelming stressors in his life. By stressors, I mean those situations that he perceives to be threatening and largely out of his control. Such stressors can include his marriage, job, or finances.

In their attempts to create security, Satiation personalities often discover that they are powerless to affect their environments and create the type of security they are looking for. About the only thing they can create is boredom. Powerlessness, low self-esteem, and boredom lead inevitably to hopelessness and depression. Ironically, despite all that they have sacrificed for a sense of safety, the Satiation-depressed personality does not experience much security, either.

A Weak Sense of Self

All of this behavior springs from an inability—perhaps even a refusal—to develop a strong sense of self. The Satiation-depressed person is aware that she lacks a set of values and convictions that are personally nurturing and defining in a positive way. Not only is she unable to say, "This is who I am," but even more fundamentally, she is unable to *feel* who she is, especially in challenging situations. This is one of the major reasons she withdraws: when faced with a challenge, the Satiation-depressed person has no anchor that would allow her to make a stand, no set of values that might serve as a compass for her actions. This inability to develop a strong senese of self is caused by the low levels of serotonin. Having low serotonin can cause a person to misperceive her self-worth and accomplishments, causing her to lose confidence or even preventing her from developing confidence. Thus, she is like a leaf in the wind, driven by the prevailing attitudes of those around her. This is not to say that she doesn't complain as she drifts along. The people-pleasing types may express their reservations (politely) and the cynics may complain bitterly (often in mocking tones) about the people leading the way, but both usually end up going along, even when they secretly believe that everyone is headed for the proverbial cliff.

The inability to experience one's true self prevents a person from defining his own needs in life. This means that he cannot define his own larger ambitions and dreams and thus cannot set a course in life. On a more immediate and practical level, the Satiation-depressed person rarely knows what he wants at any given moment and thus is rarely if ever satisfied. This leads many Satiation-depressed people to expect others to define their needs—a task at which their friends and colleagues inevitably fail. Those friends who try to comply with this unstated request to satisfy the needs of their depressed friend are, in fact, entering into a codependent relationship in which neither party will be happy or fulfilled.

Satiation-depressed people inevitably regret their past actions and criticize themselves mercilessly. The road behind them is littered with their failures, at least the way they interpret things. Hence, they are plagued by feelings of inadequacy. The primary cause of this condition is low serotonin, the chemical that is responsible for providing us with feelings of self-worth and high self-esteem.

This self-criticism also springs from their penchant for measuring themselves against unrealistic ideals. In this way, Satiation-depressed people set themselves up for failure. "I should have done this" or "I should have done that" are common refrains of the Satiation-depressed person. For some, their lofty ideals are mixed with religious beliefs that fuel feelings of self-condemnation.

Such an outlook on life promotes perfectionism, which can be one of the short roads to depression. Perfectionism is often fueled by high ideals that in actuality cannot be met. Thus, even when the person's accomplishments are significant, she thinks she has failed.

This brings me to another common characteristic of Satiation-depressed people: no matter how much they have accomplished in life or how dearly they want to be loved, they cannot bear the praise of others and usually turn such praise into its opposite in their own minds. The minute some well-intentioned person offers a compliment or praise, the Satiation-depressed person dismisses it as empty of any real meaning. He says to himself something like "My boss didn't really mean it; she only praised me to be nice," or "I didn't really do as good a job as they're saying. Actually, I did a lousy job and it's just a matter of time before they discover that I'm not so good. They'll all hate me in a few weeks." In such cases, the Satiation-depressed person uses unrealistic ideals to destroy what could have been an esteem-boosting experience. In the end, they cannot enjoy their talents or accomplishments.

The irony is that Satiation-type people, including those who are depressed, desperately want to be respected for what they do. Often they work exceptionally hard—even overwork—to gain respect and appreciation from their colleagues. Yet no matter how good a job they do or how hard they work, they rarely if ever honor their own talent and competence or fully appreciate their own contribution to the job or collective endeavor. This, of course, only contributes to their underlying insecurity.

The insistence that ideals are the only measure of their value is further evidence of their lack of a strong sense of self and their inability to nurture themselves. Satiation-depressed people have nowhere to go inside themselves that is compassionate, understanding, and nurturing.

One of the most common ways Satiation-depressed people gain relief from their self-condemnation is to indulge in short-term serotonin boosting by turning to refined sugar, carbohydrates, alcohol, or drugs to escape their own inner turmoil. Another common way is to blame others for their travails. They bitterly hold grudges—sometimes for many years—and try to make others responsible for the condition of their own lives.

Whether they are using addiction or blame, Satiation-depressed people are really trying to escape the awesome burden they carry on their shoulders. They have the feeling that they are powerless to create a positive future and therefore are marked by fate for misfortune.

These very characteristics lead some Satiation-depressed people into the kind of psychotherapy that allows them to talk endlessly about their difficulties but does not challenge them to change. This is exactly what the person secretly wants. Many therapists believe that their clients must come to their own solutions and begin to adopt new behaviors on their own. However, because challenge and change promote uncomfortable levels of norepinephrine and dopamine, Satiation types do all they can to avoid change. In the end, passive forms of therapy maintain the Satiation-depressed person's brain chemistry in exactly the way that supports the depression, which means that the therapy is not only expensive but worthless.

Joe's Recovery

The first thing I had Joe do was change his way of eating and start exercising. Satiation types usually adhere well to dietary change, but they often resist exercise. Exercise raises norepinephrine and dopamine temporarily, which many Satiation types find stressful at first. Yet exercise also raises serotonin levels and improves one's overall sense of strength and well-being. So I had Joe adopt a diet that was rich in whole grains and whole-grain products (see Chapters Seven and Eight for diets for Satiation personalities). I also encouraged him strongly to avoid refined grains and especially sugar. In addition, I urged him to do twenty minutes of stretching exercises each day for one month.

As expected, Joe dramatically increased his intake of grains and avoided sugar, and he found himself feeling stronger as a result. He also did his daily stretching routines, which were not at all strenuous. These boosted serotonin as well. After a month, I increased Joe's exercise to include brisk walking four times per week. This was all the exercise he had to do. As I explained to Joe, one of the benefits of exercise is that it quickly raises our tolerance levels for norepinephrine and dopamine. Even though exercise raises both of these gas-pedal neurotransmitters, it also gives us a physical outlet for the feelings of stress they create. In the process, a remarkable sense of personal power begins to grow. We feel stress, but we also feel ourselves doing something about it. In this way, exercise alters our brain chemistry and has a direct impact on our sense of self and personal power. Anyone who has adopted an exercise program and maintained it knows firsthand how much it increases one's sense of personal accomplishment. This is exactly what happened to Joe.

Meanwhile, I had him start writing down his feelings in a journal each day. I asked him to write for a minimum of ten minutes, and as often as he could, he should extend the time as much as possible. I also urged him to listen mostly to Satiation music every day but to add regular doses of Arousal music as a balance.

All of these factors had a profound effect on Joe. On his own he chose to start seeing a counselor once a week. Recently Joe told me that he no longer suffered from chronic depression, that he was still on the program I gave him, and that his therapy was going well. He had also entered into a new relationship.

➤ Are You a Satiation-Depressed Person?

By now you probably have guessed whether you are a Satiation-depressed person or not. The following questionnaire will help you identify the specific issues facing you and determine whether this is indeed the type of depression you experience. If you answer "yes" to more than half of these questions, chances are good that you do suffer some degree of Satiation depression.

1. Do you find yourself struggling with low energy?
2. Do you find yourself consumed regularly by negative thoughts about particular people or situations?
3. Do you criticize yourself routinely, perhaps even on a daily basis?
4. Do you believe that life does not offer many rewards?
5. Do you believe that you are not sufficiently respected, appreciated, and rewarded in your relationships?
6. Do you believe that people take you for granted?
7. Do you have trouble accepting compliments?
8. In general, do you struggle with feelings of inadequacy?
9. Do you feel that everything you do has to be perfect in order for your work or efforts to be rewarded?
10. Do you fantasize about being part of a group where everyone likes you?

Four Steps to Healing Satiation Depression

Satiation depression can be alleviated and overcome through the following four major steps. These steps are discussed in detail in Chapter Eight.

STEP ONE

The first step is to begin to recognize how your imbalanced brain chemistry has created a set of misperceptions that have become your belief system. In other words, your imbalanced brain chemistry is giving rise to thoughts and behaviors that represent a one-sided approach to life. This approach is cutting you off from certain health-promoting activities that would relieve your symptoms and promote a greater sense of personal power, identity, and freedom. The irony is that you fear behaviors that will, in fact, be medicinal for your condition.

STEP TWO

The second step is to adopt the brain-chemistry model for your personality type in order to balance your neurochemistry. Specifically, you will need to boost serotonin levels while gradually increasing norepinephrine and your tolerance for excitement and arousal. Both of these goals are accomplished through the use of a variety of health-promoting methods, including appropriate diet, exercise, and other activities. (These are described in detail in Chapter Eight.)

STEP THREE

The third step is to begin to develop a stronger sense of self by experiencing your feelings. Methods for identifying and experiencing your feelings are described in Part Two. Here is a summary of the approach I recommend:

1. Make a list of your most important needs and desires. Examples of commonly felt needs among Satiation personalities include

   > I want to feel important.
   >
   > I want to be rewarded for my work.
   >
   > I want to make a difference in the lives of others.
   >
   > I need a sense of purpose in life.
   >
   > I need to give of myself.
   >
   > I need to be heard by others and respected for what I say.
   >
   > I need to feel safe.
   >
   > I need to be able to be wrong without being made to feel ashamed or guilty.
   >
   > I need to be able to feel right and acknowledged for being right.

I need to be desirable.

I need to have my opinions considered.

I need to laugh.

I need to feel joy.

I need to express myself.

I need to grieve the losses I have experienced in my life.

I need to acknowledge fears and anger.

I need privacy and quiet time.

I need to feel hope (which is a big serotonin booster).

2. Begin to ask for your needs and desires to be met.

STEP FOUR

The fourth step is to confront your problem situations, or stressors, directly but at a rate that will not overwhelm you. This will gradually boost your levels of norepinephrine and your tolerance for this gas-pedal brain chemical. This, in turn, will increase your tolerance for excitement and arousing situations. Finally, it will boost your sense of self, personal power, and security.

This step includes the use of sleep management techniques to increase norepinephrine. Low serotonin and low norepinephrine are associated with the desire for more sleep, which is a common characteristic of Satiation-depressed people. You may lack willpower and feel the need to retreat from life; sleep is often used as an escape. Interestingly, research has shown that among some depressed people, sleep management—that is, a reduction in the number of hours they sleep—causes a significant elevation of mood. Using the brain-chemistry model, we can see that sleep management would work for Satiation-depressed people. Sleep causes temporary increases in serotonin but a diminution of norepinephrine and dopamine, neurochemicals that are needed for muscle and nervous system activity, both of which are quieted during sleep. By reducing the number of hours you sleep, you will be gently increasing norepinephrine and dopamine, thus increasing your feelings of alertness, strength, and energy. The absence of these very feelings contributes to the despair that characterizes Satiation depression.

Common Characteristics of the Satiation-Depressed Person

The following list briefly summarizes the feelings and behaviors that are common to people with this type of depression. These descriptions have been simplified and exaggerated to make it easy to see how these beliefs and behaviors help create depression.

They experience low self-worth.

They cannot accept compliments. Typically they deny the sincerity of compliments or insist that they are unworthy of praise, appreciation, and even love.

They fear becoming egocentric.

They have strong feelings of inadequacy.

"I am worthless" is a common statement they make to themselves.

They lack purpose yet deeply need a sense of direction in life.

They indulge in short-term avoidance of pain and stress.

They rarely experience accomplishment, pleasure, and joy.

They experience internal rewards for the avoidance of pain rather than the experience of pleasure.

They are filled with shame, guilt, and conflict.

They do not believe they deserve the blessings of life.

They control situations and others through the avoidance of conflict and through passivity, weakness, and compliance.

They seek to maintain the status quo.

They are procrastinators.

They eat compulsively.

They often spend compulsively.

They are often codependent and create relationships based on an implicit agreement: "I will not tell on you if you do not tell on me; I will not define your problem if you do not define mine."

They expect others to define their needs.

Since they never define or clarify their own needs, these needs are never met.

They want sympathy, because sympathy keeps people from having to change.

They join groups that will sustain their picture of themselves and of reality.

They find safety in the absence of stimuli.

They escape from demands.

They feel they were born to fail. "I was made imperfect and worthless; it's God's fault."

They are not able to ask for help.

If you are a Satiation-depressed person, you need a sense of purpose that will take you out of yourself—but before you can venture forth, you need to change your brain chemistry in order to feel capable of entering the unknown. The tools and the program described in Chapters Seven and Eight will help you to do exactly that.

Chapter 5

The Arousal-Depressed Personality

Nancy is a forty-year-old mother of two, with a good marriage and a very demanding career as a social worker. She is extremely competent at her job, as in all other areas of her life. She is the kind of woman people depend on to meet their needs. She wants very much to do good at the same time that she is doing well. She loves her children and husband and cares deeply for her clients, who relate to her almost as if they were her children. In short, the demands of her life are overwhelming, and she must push herself hard to meet them. As she says, "I spend a lot of days running after myself." In order to maintain her frenetic pace, she drinks a lot of coffee, eats considerable amounts of red meat, especially as fast food, and maintains a high level of anxiety. Not surprisingly, she suffers from a variety of health problems—namely, menstrual irregularities, digestive disorders, and pain in her chest. Periodically, she experiences what she can only describe as a "panic attack," meaning she is overwhelmed by all the possible things that could go wrong in any given day. Many of her days are driven by some kind of crisis. She lives under constant stress.

Recently, she got the flu and was forced to rest for several days. The break from her routine was "horrible," she says. "I was depressed the entire time. I don't know why, but I felt horrible. I sank like a stone, and the longer I was away from the job, the worse it got." Even before she was fully well, she was back at the job, pushing herself relentlessly. She admits that this cycle recurs whenever she gets sick. Even she has some vague intimation that "the big one"—some kind of major health crisis—may lie ahead of her unless she changes her ways. Until she came to me, however, she had no idea how she could change the pace of her life.

The problem Nancy faces is that beneath her anxiety lies a depression that she refuses to confront. She uses stress and anxiety to keep herself from feeling her depression. As long as her life is overwhelmed by demands and crises, she manages to keep her focus on the present moment and away from her inner condition. Still, as everyone knows, anxiety, crisis, and stress have serious side effects, not the least of which is their negative impact on physical health.

Nancy suffers from what I call Arousal depression, a type common among many inordinately active men and women.

Arousal Depression: Excitement as Medication

The Arousal-depressed person typically has relatively low to extremely low brain levels of serotonin, coupled with relatively high to extremely high levels of norepinephrine and dopamine. This combination of chemicals causes the person to feel that life is continually out of control and heading for disaster. He must somehow control events in order to keep from experiencing terrible failure and collapse. Of course, when one has to control events constantly, one's inner life is dominated by anxiety.

The anxiety of the Arousal-depressed person, in fact, masks her depression. If you ask people who suffer from Arousal depression what they feel when they relax and allow themselves to experience their inner state, the answers you will hear most often include "worried," "stressed," "anxious," "nervous," "pressured," "tense," "harassed," "overworked," tired," and "afraid." These adjectives actually describe just their first layer of feeling. Arousal-depressed people rarely know that below their anxiety lies a deep and abiding depression. This depression only surfaces when they are sick, or bored, or trapped in a situation that they cannot change. Hence, they avoid at all costs any situation that will constrain them or force them to feel their underlying feelings.

In order to avoid such conditions, Arousal-depressed people are always in motion. They fill up their lives with deadlines, people, demands, and exercise routines. They are action-oriented and constantly on the go. They live fast-paced lives with lots of stimulation. They prefer jobs that allow them to get out of the office and force them to drive in traffic and rush to closely scheduled appointments that are at opposite ends of the city.

All this activity and pressure promotes the production of norepinephrine and dopamine, and these neurotransmitters in turn increase both these people's anxiety and their capacity to deal with many different kinds of demands and constant change. But the high anxiety also keeps them from feeling the one thing that they are truly terrified of: their depression. Thus, Arousal-depressed people use their fast-paced lifestyle and high anxiety as a form of medication to keep them from experiencing the feelings that lie beneath all the tension and fear. Not surprisingly, any inactivity or slowdown in the pace of their lives is extremely uncomfortable for Arousal-depressed people. In fact, they will go to great lengths to avoid such a slowdown, even creating crises in their jobs or their personal lives in order to avoid feeling their latent depression. If things begin to slow down or get boring, they'll move, or change jobs, or break off relationships—anything to keep from feeling their own pain.

I am not saying that every active person is depressed. Depression is usually the result of a one-sided personality, whether it be a Satiation or an Arousal type. People avoid depression by achieving a balance between the two, which is reflected in their balanced brain chemistries. If a person is exceedingly active but also enjoys Satiation activities—especially intimacy with himself and others—he is much more likely to have a healthy and balanced Arousal personality.

One of the common characteristics of depression is sleep disorder. Very often, the combination of low serotonin and high norepinephrine and dopamine prevent deep and restful sleep in the Arousal-depressed person. Serotonin, you will recall, is essential for deep sleep. It is a mellowing chemical and allows the person to relax and let go of the day's events. People with relatively low serotonin often have trouble getting to sleep, and they tend to experience shallow sleep from which they are easily awakened. By not sleeping deeply, they never become fully rested. In addition, sleep is essential to psychological and physical health. During sleep, the immune system is strengthened and the body is able to heal itself. Those who do not get adequate sleep often suffer from weakened immune systems, as well as a range of psychological imbalances, such as further anxiety, increasing fear and insecurities, and misperceptions.

Arousal depression usually causes inadequate sleep, while Satiation depression is often associated with too much sleep. This difference is caused by the brain-chemistry configuration associated with each type. In Arousal depression, the low serotonin and high norepinephrine cause the person to remain alert, active, and awake for long hours. In Satiation depression, the low serotonin and low norepinephrine combine to create a desire to escape from reality by sleeping more.

Control at All Costs

Control is an issue for both Satiation- and Arousal-depressed people. We tend to turn to control when we feel out of balance. The control from the Satiation-depressed person tends to be passive-aggressive. These people are prone to perfectionism, cleaning, and using guilt as forms of control. Although Arousal-depressed people may also use similar behaviors, they are more likely to be aggressive. They might manipulate facts, people, and situations and use blame to get what they want.

High levels of norepinephrine increase the rate of neurotransmission, which heightens alertness and speeds up a person's thoughts and words. Other characteristics related to high norepinephrine include enhanced assertiveness, rapid physical reactions, aggression, and a strong desire to speed up events or control them. This might describe a strong leader if it were not for the fact that the low serotonin usually creates low self-esteem, low self-confidence, and too much fear about what other people are thinking. As I discussed in Chapter Two, animal studies have shown that leaders are characteristically high in serotonin; the animals on the lower rungs of the social ladder typically are low in serotonin and high in norepinephrine and dopamine. These animals are not only anxious but often violent. Research on humans has shown that high levels of norepinephrine and dopamine increase the likelihood of violent behavior, including against oneself. It seems that this brain-chemistry combination—especially when serotonin is very low and norepinephrine and dopamine very high—gives rise not only to violence but to self-hatred. This type of brain-chemistry imbalance also causes confused or chaotic thinking. The vast majority of Arousal-depressed people are not at all violent, but they do lack the self-confidence and self-esteem to relax, concentrate on the issues at hand, and lead people in a balanced and methodical manner.

The combination of anxiety, rapid neurotransmission, and enhanced aggression creates a personality that seeks to control the future in order to avoid disaster. Arousal-depressed people are universally focused outside themselves. They cannot bear to look within. They measure the relative safety of their lives based on information they get from the environment—that is, on the behavior of their friends, loved ones, coworkers, and employers. They are highly sensitive and vulnerable to the information they receive from others. Their moods rise and fall based on what others are saying about them today or on the outcome of their latest challenge or travail. Many—but certainly not all—type A individuals are Arousal personalities who are depressed.

Of course, such characteristics make for a person who is extremely goal-oriented and highly competitive. These people try to control their environments to get what they want. Unfortunately, the more one tries to control the future and the outside world, the more anxiety one suffers. Thus, Arousal-depressed people usually overwork, overworry, and overcontrol situations. They expend enormous amounts of energy on everything they do, usually putting out much more energy than is actually needed to succeed in the situation. Consequently, Arousal-depressed people are not only depressed but exhausted. As with their depression, they medicate their exhaustion with more norepinephrine and dopamine, both of which provide additional energy. They push themselves with caffeine and nervous tension, in part because rest is terrifying to them. Rest, after all, will cause them to feel their feelings, including their depression.

Beneath the comparisons and competition, however, is a person who yearns to be admired yet fears being different in any negative sense. The Arousal-depressed person wants to be appreciated for her uniqueness. She wants to be acknowledged for the amount of effort she is putting out, because secretly she longs to be irreplaceable and essential to others. She longs to have the world depend on her, because this will ensure the kind of security she needs.

Arousal-depressed people need lots of compliments and stroking in order to feel comfortable, especially in situations that are foreign. They need to be reassured that their own lofty image of themselves is held by others. This need, of course, reveals how insecure they are and how much they doubt themselves.

Usually an Arousal-depressed person measures how much he is needed or admired through his material possessions and other forms of status—a lofty job title, a big house, or the corner office. In contrast to Satiation-depressed people, Arousal-depressed people think that they have identified their needs—but they are rarely accurate. What they have identified is their need for status and admiration from the outside world, which are often some of life's most ephemeral rewards.

Since they are externally directed, Arousal-depressed people usually blame others for their problems. The prospect of being identified and singled out as the cause of a problem is one of the most terrifying thoughts they can have. This situation would force them to focus on the depression and isolation they feel deep within. It's very hard to show an Arousal-depressed person that she is wrong in a particular circumstance. Like other extreme type A personalities, they measure their self-worth solely on achievement. Achieving success, being good, and being right are essential to survival. Therefore, they are brilliant at justifying themselves, rationalizing their behavior, and finding some external crisis on which to focus.

Needless to say, Arousal-depressed people have great difficulty with all forms of intimacy, especially intimacy with themselves. They like to keep things light, superficial, and fun. Don't become too serious around an Arousal-depressed person; he'll be out the door before you complete the sentence. This makes things very difficult in a marriage. It eliminates a lot of activities, situations, and settings that the spouse of the Arousal-depressed person might enjoy sharing.

Not surprisingly, Arousal-depressed people often marry someone who is equally uncomfortable with her feelings, which protects the Arousal personality from being confronted with a lot of issues emerging from his underlying depression. The minute a spouse starts to demand more intimacy or quiet time, the Arousal-depressed person usually finds something to do: he leaves the room to catch up on some paperwork or starts building an addition to the house.

The Abyss

The danger for Arousal-depressed people is that their gas-pedal chemicals may get so high that they will begin to suffer from paranoia and delusion. When norepinephrine and dopamine become exceedingly high—as can be the case when a person is pushing himself way too hard—he can become irrationally insecure and even paranoid about those around him. In effect, he projects his own darkest thoughts and fears onto his coworkers, spouse, and friends. The world is against him, he thinks. The only way to deal with this is to become more aggressive, more controlling, and ultimately to fight back. This, of course, can lead a person to feel even more overwhelmed, oppressed, and weakened by all that he must face in life. "No one understands me," the Arousal-depressed person says. But rather than back away and allow the situation to cool, the Arousal-depressed person often tries even harder to make things right, usually controlling the events to his detriment.

Some Arousal-depressed people who are pushed to their limit find their way into drug addiction, especially to amphetamines and specifically to cocaine. Cocaine raises dopamine and norepinephrine levels instantly, causing a rapid increase in neurotransmission and giving the person the illusion of being in control. With the elevation in neurotransmission comes greater lucidity, enhanced language skills, and increased physical coordination. One of the major problems with cocaine, of course, is that its associated "high" is short-lived, and the fall from its drug-induced heights is dramatic. Norepinephrine and dopamine levels plummet from the extremely high elevations caused by the drug to below-normal levels. For the Arousal personality who is already depressed, the resulting depression is severe. All she can feel at this point is the depression caused by low serotonin in combination with low dopamine and norepinephrine. The only way to escape this wasteland is to consume more cocaine. Again, her brain chemistry takes a roller-coaster ride, but it too can only end in despair. In a very short time, the body's ability to sustain its baseline of elevated norepinephrine and dopamine is weakened, because these elevations have been caused by an outside, artificial substance—namely, cocaine. Unable to bear the low brain levels of norepinephrine and dopamine and the related depression, the person is forced to rely even more heavily on cocaine; this is the cycle of addiction.

➤ Are You an Arousal-Depressed Person?

This description has probably allowed you to guess whether or not you suffer from Arousal depression. The following questionnaire will help you identify the specific issues facing you and determine whether this is indeed the type of depression you experience. If you answer "yes" to more than half of these questions, chances are good that you do suffer some degree of Arousal depression.

1. Do you find yourself feeling that if only things or people were different you'd be just fine?

2. Do you often feel that you know what is best for others?

3. When you get into a conflict in a relationship, do you get frustrated when the other person doesn't follow your advice?

4. Do you find yourself able to justify most of your actions, and do you believe you are right in virtually every case?

5. Do you blame others for situations that go wrong in your life?

6. Do you have a strong fear of failure?

7. Do you find that others don't meet your expectations?

8. Do you get frustrated because others do not notice your uniqueness or the uniqueness of your contribution to a given endeavor?

9. Do you find that others do not understand you?

10. Do you use sex, alcohol, or drugs to reduce anxiety, frustration, or fear?

11. Do you have trouble relaxing or enjoying intimate environments or conversations?

12. Do you avoid conversations or change the subject when people start to confess their troubles, personal struggles, or failures?

13. Do you avoid revealing your weaknesses, vulnerabilities, or doubts to others?

14. Do you wish you could tell someone your fears, doubts, and vulnerabilities without losing that person's respect or admiration?

Four Steps to Healing Arousal Depression

With this bird's-eye view of the characteristics of a person with Arousal depression, we can easily see that the problems stem mostly from the extreme one-sidedness of the personality and the strategies the person uses to get through life. Obviously, the person caught up in Arousal depression feels that she is doing everything she must do to survive. She believes that if she were to stop trying to control everything, her world would fall apart. So simply advising this person to relax, or slow down, or take a different approach to life is useless, though well-meaning friends and relatives probably offer such advice endlessly. What people must realize is that slowing down and letting life take its course are the very things that terrify the Arousal-depressed personality and that drive much of her behavior.

The most effective approach to healing Arousal depression involves the following four major steps. A complete program for overcoming this type of depression is offered in Chapter Nine.

STEP ONE
If you are an Arousal-depressed person, you first need to adopt the brain-chemistry model for your personality type and begin to raise serotonin levels and lower dopamine and norepinephrine levels. Changing your perceptions and behavior will be much easier as serotonin increases and norepinephrine decreases. This change in brain chemistry alone will boost feelings of well-being, confidence, and enhanced self-esteem, while at the same time reducing anxiety, nervous tension, and fear.

STEP TWO
The second step is simply to question your belief system without doing anything to change it. All you must do, at least at first, is to open up to the *possibility* that there is another way to live. I want to empha-

size that you do not have to change anything—not until you feel you *want* to change. Changing your behavior will come after your brain chemistry has become more balanced. But before such changes can take place, you must begin to feel comfortable with the idea of change and to recognize that it isn't dangerous. Such an attitude will support the changes you are making in your brain chemistry and will allow your transformation to occur more quickly.

STEP THREE

Allow yourself to experience the feelings that exist beneath your anxiety. This must be accomplished gradually, in small digestible amounts. I recommend short periods of prayer or meditation in which you focus on what you actually feel, as opposed to what you think you should feel. I also recommend checking in with your feelings during those times of the day when you are ordinarily unconscious of your inner state, such as when you get into the car to drive to work or run an errand, when you sit down at your desk, or when you're on your way home from the job. Practice turning your focus inward and recognizing the feelings you are experiencing. Do not try to change or repress what you feel. Rather, honor your feelings and develop compassion for yourself.

One way to become more self-reflective and aware of your feelings is to experience how it feels when you:

- Stop teaching or providing answers to others. What happens when you give yourself permission to ask questions, be receptive, and learn?

- Seek to establish balance in your life by taking care of your needs. What do you feel when you are quiet or alone, or take time to self-reflect?

- Shift your focus from goals to the daily process that leads to your goals. What would life be like if there were no goals to accomplish and all that mattered was your daily quality of life?

- Become more aware of the needs of those close to you. How does it feel to give attention to others without having any agenda or secret goals in mind?

STEP FOUR

Recognize that you have a vast array of needs that are currently going unmet. You have a need to be quiet and to be receptive—not only to others but to yourself. You have a need to be safe without having to create that safety yourself. You have a need to be supported. You have a need to relax. You have a strong need to free yourself from judgment—your own as well as that of others. You have a need to give without expecting anything in return, just as you need to receive without feeling that you owe anything to anyone. You have a strong need to feel humble, grateful, and compassionate toward yourself.

Becoming aware of your needs is the first step toward fulfilling them. As you become more aware of your needs, you will find a deeper satisfaction and fulfillment and joy than can be experienced in any other way.

Common Characteristics of the Arousal-Depressed Person

The following list briefly summarizes the feelings and behaviors that are common to people with this type of depression. These descriptions have been simplified and exaggerated to make it easy to see how these beliefs and behaviors help create depression.

They suffer from low self-esteem, yet often don't know it.

They want to be admired by others; they want others to support and reinforce their own best image of themselves.

They often believe that the end justifies the means.

They attempt to control people and their environment.

They have unrealistic expectations of others because they need so much support from the environment.

Their expectations are usually focused on coworkers, boss, wife, family, and God.

Many suffer from deep anger and bitterness, which can be focused on others or on themselves.

They believe that the outside environment must serve them—everyone else has to change; they do not have to change.

They attempt to make themselves indispensable to others, especially to spouse, company, employer, and friends.

They need to be on top of the heap in order to feel safe.

They strive so hard to be needed and wanted that they expend enormous amounts of energy.

They want everyone to see their uniqueness; this ensures safety and success because it ensures that they are needed.

They need lots of applause and compliments in order to feel secure.

When confronted with criticism, they blame others, including the person doing the criticizing.

They feel it is essential to be right, to know the answers.

They are given to grandiosity, especially in private moments or in talking about personal matters with others.

They become deeply disenchanted with others who do not recognize them.

Their love is conditioned on getting the kind of feedback and praise they desire.

They have an innate need to evaluate another person's love. They constantly ask, "Are they loving me enough?"

Their implicit agreement with their spouse and close relationship is "Love me for what I do for you."

They want to be seen as essential to any task they take on.

They are highly vulnerable to criticism and changes of attitude from people around them.

They feel that no one understands them, even God.

They feel they are never really appreciated, no matter what they do.

Their basic problem is their refusal to be open to another way of being or to another perspective on a situation.

They often intellectualize feelings and problems to justify their behavior.

They are frequently workaholics.

They often enjoy alcohol, including hard liquors.

They can be compulsive spenders.

They are risk takers.

They can be promiscuous as a way to avoid feelings, relationships, and intimacy with others and self.

They frequently feel cheated or angry, and they have deep resentments.

They do things to reward themselves in order to compensate for the unfairness of the world.

They are very competitive and constantly compare themselves with others.

They control others through aggression.

If you are an Arousal-depressed person, you need to have a sense of purpose that includes others and their intimacy and your true needs—but before you can venture forth, you need to change your brain chemistry in order to see yourself, others, and God less conditionally. The tools and the program described in Chapters Seven and Nine will help you do exactly that.

Chapter 6

Trigger Situations

I can't figure it out," Glenda said. "I'm doing so well and then, bang! I get depressed. If only I could stop it—you know, see it coming."

"You can do that," I answered. "You can see it coming and stop it, too."

"Oh, sure. All I need is a crystal ball and a drawer full of uppers."

"No, you can do it without drugs," I said. "Not even coffee or colas."

"I don't think that's possible." But as Glenda said these words, her eyes revealed something else. It was a glimmer—not much more than a trace—of hope. Up to that point, she had been taking anti-depressants for three years. As far as Glenda was concerned, she had tried everything and failed.

"Do you know how a gun works?" I asked. When she nodded, I said, "You can't fire unless you pull the trigger, right? Well, your brain works the same way. Your depressive reaction can't begin without a stimulus, a trigger. What if you could learn how *not* to pull the trigger? What if you could stop the depressive reaction before it happens?"

Glenda leaned forward, her silence begging me to explain more. That's when I told her about what I call triggers—the automatic feelings or situations that set off your depression. These triggers don't *cause* your depression, but they are *associated* with it. They are the device that leads you into depression. At some point in your life, you were conditioned to respond to a stimulus in a certain way, and this response creates a chemical imbalance in the brain. This imbalance causes you to perceive reality inaccurately and to misinterpret events around you. Let me repeat: every time you respond to this stimulus—every time you "pull the trigger"—your brain chemistry becomes unbalanced and you get depressed. Then you have to do something to restore balance. Some people reach for drugs. Others accept their depression as inevitable and live in misery. But even if the trigger for your depression seems to come without warning, you can learn to recognize it. And if you learn to understand your triggers, you can stop the response before it happens.

The Concept of the Conditioned Response

Ivan P. Pavlov (1849–1936) was a Russian physiologist who first discovered the workings of digestion, but he is now famous for demonstrating how the mind can be conditioned to respond to a repeated experience. Many people know of his experiments with dogs, which led to what is sometimes called conditioned behavior—a method that causes natural responses of the glands or muscles (automatic, unconscious behavior) to be brought on by stimuli that would not ordinarily have any effect. His experiment was built around the innate or unconditioned reflex of salivation in response to meat in the mouth. This response occurs in all animals, including humans. Pavlov reasoned that if the animals began to associate getting food with something else, such as a circle of light or the sound of a bell, eventually the sight or the sound alone would cause salivation. In his experiments, every time the animals received meat, they heard a bell ring. Pavlov and his assistants repeated this combination again and again. Once Pavlov believed that the animals had associated the sound of the bell with getting food, he moved on to the next phase of the experiment. Now he rang the bell but provided no food. Regardless of whether the animals saw food or not, as soon as they heard that particular bell, they salivated. It became an automatic response.

Pavlov's experiment provided the foundation for our understanding of what we call *conditioned behavior* in human beings and other animals. In conditioned behavior, an activity that is normally voluntary, or under conscious control, becomes automatic and unconscious. With an automatic or conditioned response, we have no choice in how we behave. We all have conditioned responses.

As a child, you were conditioned every time you responded to a conflict in a certain way and got a reward. For example, if you felt like you had let your parents down, perhaps by getting a poor grade or by not doing something right, and if you found that having a piece of candy and going for a walk made you feel better, you began to develop a conditioned response. After enough repetitions of the stimulus and reward, you began to respond automatically to conflict by wanting to go off by yourself and eat sweets.

Depressed people develop a set of conditioned responses that tell them to feel depressed. These responses occur in association with what I call *triggers*—stimuli that set off your depression. Like Pavlov's dogs, you don't reason out that you've only heard the bell and there is no meat in sight; you just respond automatically with depression. Understanding your triggers is vital to overcoming your depression. Although we have responses other than depression, such as eating or smoking, we will focus on depression in this book.

I'll give you a simple illustration of depression as a conditioned response. Sally is a middle-aged woman who came to me for treatment of her depression. She had been abused by her father. All the men she dated were abusive types who treated her badly. She then married an alcoholic who was verbally abusive. She divorced him and decided to try marriage again, but at this point depression hit her hard.

She wanted a relationship, yet every time she thought about a new relationship, she got depressed. She had developed a conditioned response. Her relationships meant pain and rejection, and these, of course, are depressing. So every time Sally even thought about relationship, she got depressed.

For a long time Sally focused on the depression itself as the cause of her problem. "Why do I feel so blue? What's wrong with me?" she asked herself time and time again. She was looking at the result instead of the stimulus that caused it. In other words, she was failing to notice the trigger that was associated with a particular response. Sally had been conditioned since childhood to believe that the search for a relationship would lead to rejection. The first time she'd had this experience was with her father, who had sexually abused her and then abandoned her. Her subsequent relationships with males had reinforced this association of relationship with rejection. Since for Sally, rejection always led to depression, eventually the mere thought of relationship could trigger depression for Sally. It's really that simple. In Sally's case, you can see the trigger because I have isolated it for you. But Sally could not see it.

Not all conditioned responses are harmful, but some are. This chapter will help you determine what triggers cause such automatic depression responses that they happen without your being aware of them. Let me give you another example. Suppose you grew up in a home where your father got angry and then your mother emotionally withdrew. She stayed depressed for days. If you observed this long enough, you may have learned this action unknowingly. If your father raged, you wilted, withdrew emotionally, and felt depressed. Because this happened often, on a level far below your consciousness, the trigger was put in place. Now whenever you hear an angry attack, you automatically become depressed. As a child, depression was your way of avoiding your lack of security or fear of bodily pain. Now it has become a conditioned response to any trigger that reminds you of that original situation.

Let's say you didn't get depressed when your father raged. Suppose you noticed that your mother reached for the aspirin bottle and complained about a headache. If you think it through, you may discover that you started on the road to looking for medicine to take away your pain because these two things became associated with each other very early in your life. Now, whenever you experience emotional pain, you try to cure it with medicine. In those early days, aggression led to emotional pain (the stimulus or *trigger*). Medication (the *response*) led to feeling better. Now you have an automatic response to medicate yourself in an emotionally painful situation. Medication, however, is not always an appropriate response to every negative feeling. In fact, medication may be causing you to feel depressed rather than helping you deal with the source of the pain.

Your behavior, such as depression, can begin as a subconscious choice—your mind chooses to feel depressed in response to pain. If this is repeated, eventually it will become an automatic response. Your ability to choose consciously not to be depressed or not to behave in a certain way is then taken away. Unconscious choices are always more powerful because we have no conscious memory of when we gave up our right to choose our actions. The secret to regaining control of your actions (and thereby preventing depression) is to become aware of what triggers these actions.

Remember, a trigger is a neutral stimulus that you habitually associate with your depression. To discover your trigger, you must look at whatever happens in your life just before the onset of depression. If you learn to recognize the trigger, you can learn healthy ways to cope instead of slipping into depression.

Step One: Identifying Your Conditioned Responses

To begin recognizing your triggers, you first need to look at your conditioned responses. Although we know the real conditioned response is depression, we often can only see the behaviors that are a result of this depression. So we may need to identify the behaviors to determine what our triggers are and understand our depression. Remember, in the case of Pavlov's dogs, the trigger was the bell, the conditioned response was to salivate. So first you should look at how you handle conflict. What do you do when you are under stress and start to feel bad? Everyone has a different way of handling conflict. Some people run away from it, some people get angry, and others eat or drink compulsively. Start keeping a notebook handy and jot down what you do after a conflict or a particularly stressful moment. You will discover certain behaviors that you engage in repeatedly. These are your conditioned behavioral responses.

When we were children, our parents provided our first examples of how to behave. They had specific ways of reacting to conflict, and their conditioned responses helped to condition us. So to understand your conditioned responses, you also need to look back at how your parents handled conflict. What did they do after a quarrel? How did they react to confrontation? These conflicts may have involved your parents' interaction with each other, with their jobs, with you, or with other stressful situations. But the point is that any behavior your parents repeated consistently may have been incorporated into your own life. To help you think about your family when you were growing up, ask yourself these questions:

1. When conflicts arose, did your parents face them?
2. Did they avoid confronting each other?
3. Was there an aura of silence around certain issues?
4. Did they argue, scream, yell, and blame, yet never resolve issues?
5. Were rage and angry voices a common part of family life?
6. Did one parent blame the other? Or blame the children, the job, politics, society, or someone else?
7. Did one of your parents use guilt or manipulation to force family members to go along with their wishes?

Don't rush through your answers. You may even want to discuss these questions with a sibling or someone who knows your family well. Unless you are extremely unusual or have a genetically based depression, your feelings of depression are almost certainly linked to the ways in which your family reacted to conflict. The conflict may have been overt, as in a direct, verbal fight between your parents, or it may have been more subtle, as in a parent's reaction to feeling insecure. How they reacted is what is important. They used some method to avoid the conflict, to find resolution, or just to feel better. You need to look carefully at what they did.

Feeling depressed and the behaviors associated with it are conditioned responses you learned as a way of coping with conflict. After a conflict arose in your family, how did your parents react? Did one of them turn to alcohol? Cigarettes? Sex? Did they become morose and moody? Simply by being part of that family system, you may well have picked up the same behavior in response to adverse circumstances. While you as an adult have different emotional conflicts from your parents, your conditioned response is likely to be the same.

Conditioned responses are what we do to make ourselves feel better. Some people's conditioned response is to clean their house, others go shopping, and still others have sex. Whatever it is you do, it makes you feel better, and "feeling better" is tied to a chemical change in the brain. It may cause a release of "excitement" chemicals like dopamine and norepinephrine, or you may get more of a satiation response to calm your anxiety. In any case, your conditioned response is not a conscious choice, and therefore every time it happens and you get the chemical reward of feeling better, it keeps you on a treadmill of "action and reaction."

Conditioned responses are also what we do when we feel good and want to feel better. In treating hundreds of patients over the years, I have noticed that the behavior that makes people feel better when they are in conflict is often what they choose to do in order to celebrate. They clean their house, go shopping, eat a certain food to excess. So the second clue to finding your conditioned responses, and thereby your triggers, is to take note of how you celebrate. When you are feeling good about something and want to feel even better, what do you do?

Step Two: Identifying Your Trigger Emotions

When you have figured out what your automatic behaviors (conditioned responses to your depression) are, you are ready to look at what causes them, your emotions.

Emotions are what actually trigger the depression that causes our behaviors. We all have conditioned responses to many emotions. You will find that the way we behave, the conditioned response, is easier to recognize than the emotion that triggers it. How you are acting (crying, overeating, running every day, and so on) may be obvious to you. What is less obvious is why. We often don't understand our emotions, and when we don't, that bell goes off without our knowing it.

Emotions affect you in all aspects of your life. They alter hormone production, change brain chemistry, and cause medical complications. Emotions can stimulate a release of chemicals in the brain that can cause depression or anxiety. These chemicals also affect our perceptions. Have you ever noticed that when you are stressed or frustrated you seem to look at everything differently? Have you ever noticed a change in the level of your self-confidence when you are stressed? These are examples of how your perceptions are changed by brain chemicals that have been activated by your emotions. What happens is that the brain memorizes negative perceptions that have been implanted either in childhood or later in life. However, the earlier they are implanted, the more significantly they affect our lives and the more difficult they are to unravel. Because they are the foundation of what we believe to be true, we often reinforce the negative perceptions with decisions we make. For example, if my parents told me that I can't speak in public and I believed it, then I'll avoid situations that may require me to speak in public. I'll also tell people I can't speak in public and continue to reinforce this misperception. The more stressed or insecure I become, the more I will avoid public speaking. To succeed in preventing depression, I must identify those "false" perceptions stored in the brain. In the example I just gave, the emotion implanted in me was one of inadequacy. My parents had told me that I didn't make sense or that what I said was stupid. I believed that to be true and concluded that I don't have anything important to say. The trigger in this case would be the feeling of inadequacy and the behavior or conditioned response would be avoidance of public speaking. I might take this further and get depressed, thinking I can't achieve my goals because of my apparent inability to speak in public.

Understanding emotions doesn't have to be painful, nor do you have to go back into your childhood and critique your parents. The process does involve slowing down and observing yourself, and then talking to a support person about your conclusions. You can also keep a journal in which you write every day about your feelings. As you talk or write about your feelings, they will begin to be more clear to you.

Emotions can be difficult to understand because of the tricks we play on ourselves to hide how we feel from ourselves and others. There are five ways that most of us hide our emotions:

Denying

Minimizing

Justifying

Blaming

Rationalizing

Denying your emotions means pretending they don't exist. Many children are raised to deny anger, for example. Let us imagine that you were taught from birth that nice people don't get angry. Now if you get angry, you either have to accept that you are a bad person or deny that you feel angry at all. Most people will choose the latter. In order to change, you must realize that your feelings (emotions) are not right or wrong — it is the action you take in response to the feeling that can be right or wrong.

Minimizing our emotions allows us to pretend that our feelings are not as deep as they really are. You tell yourself "things aren't really that bad." For example, you may feel sad and fearful of your own death when your aging grandfather dies after a long illness that caused him a great deal of pain. Your emotion is one of grief, yet you minimize this by saying it was best for him and he is better off. You don't allow yourself to grieve because you minimize your sadness.

Justifying an emotion is a tricky way to avoid dealing with it. For example, let's say that you are angry with your parents for the way they treated you. When you think about them, you continue to build up a case against them. You prove to yourself over and over that your anger is legitimate, which only perpetuates your anger. Often we need to talk with our parents, children, siblings, or others to ask them how they saw the situation. We ask questions to try to determine the accuracy of our perceptions, not to see if our feelings are wrong. Feelings exist, yet perceptions can magnify them and cause us to create greater or different feelings that don't allow us to heal. Often a more accurate understanding of our feelings is the beginning of the healing process.

Blaming someone for an emotion is another way we avoid learning from it. Blaming others for a negative feeling we are experiencing seems to bring relief from emotional pain. Unfortunately, assigning responsibility to someone else for your emotion leaves you powerless to change your response. You must accept responsibility for your own emotions if you want to control your conditioned responses. In this way, you can take a negative feeling that previously would have triggered a depressive response and turn it into a personal challenge to make yourself stronger and happier.

Rationalizing your emotions is the big gun, your emotional elephant rifle, that keeps from facing your emotions. We rationalize away our feelings, using rationalization alone or combining it with one or more of the preceding techniques. We tell ourselves that our pain isn't there, isn't that important anyway, is really justified by someone else's actions, in fact, is really someone else's fault, and therefore is something we don't have to feel. If you are good enough at it, you can get friends, family, even your therapist to rationalize with you. Just remember, if you don't know what you are feeling, you can't change it, and the bell still rings.

Step Three: Identifying Your Trigger Situations

Two types of people come to see me for help with depression. One type says, "Doc, I'm in pain; please take it away," and the other says, "Doc, I'm in pain; what can I do to take it away?" Only those who are or who become the second type—those who learn to accept responsibility for their own emotions—ever achieve personal peace and freedom from depression. The first step in keeping your bell from ringing is to become familiar with your conditioned responses. The second step is to recognize your true emotions, especially the ones that trigger depression. The third step is to discover the situations in which those emotions arise.

Let me give you an example of the importance of recognizing your trigger situations. Matt was a hardworking, highly motivated young man. He worked as a CPA for a large accounting firm. He had been married for about three years when he recognized that he was beginning to have mood swings. Sometimes he went into such depressed moods that it really scared him. As Matt began to understand his triggers, he became aware of a connection he had never made before: whenever he faced any conflict with his wife, he became depressed. Then he dug deeper. He realized that when he was growing up, his parents had never seemed to argue with one another—no disagreements, no angry words. When Matt married and a disagreement arose, he felt rejected and inadequate. "I felt that I just wasn't much of a husband if I had to have conflict," he said. According to his upbringing, mature, intelligent, kind people did not have conflicts or disagreements. But he had strong disagreements with his wife, so something must be wrong with him. Matt learned that the trigger in his life was situational: whenever he had a disagreement with his wife, he plunged into depression.

What situations cause you to go into depression? The emotions you identified in Step Two cause your bell to ring, leading to depression. Remember that depression does not necessarily have to be the "downer" type. Depending on your brain chemistry, you may have an anxious or "arousal" type of depressive response instead. In either case, certain situations elicit your emotional triggers. Step Three involves learning what those situations are.

In general, most of us find it easier to identify our "uncomfortable" situations than we do our emotions. Nevertheless, there are several ways we try to hide from those situations in order to protect ourselves.

Avoidance. Avoiding uncomfortable situations altogether is a frequent tactic. What seems like a reasonable decision not to put yourself in a stressful situation may actually be a way of avoiding a confrontation with one of your triggers. For example, Bob, one of my clients, had broken off all contact with his father because he felt his father was very controlling and dominant. Avoiding his father because it brought up painful emotions, however, did not solve the problem. Bob still experienced the emotions of loneliness and powerlessness, but until he stopped avoiding the relationship, he didn't make the connection. As I have said, if you want to be in control of your life, you must accept your feelings without judgment. Avoiding a confrontation keeps you from changing your conditioned response into a conscious choice of action.

Manipulation. The typical response to a situation that makes us uncomfortable is to try to change it. What's wrong with this response? There may be nothing wrong, but often it masks an attempt to manipulate the circumstances and thereby avoid the problem. Remember your goal is not to make your life seem more comfortable but rather to gain conscious control of the trigger emotions that ring your bell and lead to depression.

One way of manipulating situations is through physical symptoms. Perhaps a stomachache, a headache, or the very popular backache keeps you from participating in a situation. There are times when we push beyond a headache to participate in an event that is worth it to us. Other times we tend to magnify the headache because it is a convenient excuse for avoiding the event. These physical symptoms get us out of the situation but still trigger the emotion. You may decline an invitation to go bowling because you have a headache (but really because you think you look stupid bowling). You have manipulated the situation, but you still experience the feelings of inadequacy.

Another way of manipulating situations is through anger. Anger is frequently used to avoid an intimate relationship in which we feel inadequate. If you pick a fight with someone, you can avoid him altogether. Once again, when you do this, you are masking your true emotions. That intimate relationship may bring up your fear of loneliness and rejection. Parents often blow up and get angry when a child does something wrong. In a fit of rage, the parent sends the child to her room instead of offering new and more appropriate behavior to the child. The feeling the parent is masking is one of inadequacy, of not knowing what to do. Anger and avoidance of relationship go hand in hand. You may feel inadequate, less worthy than another, or less desirable than someone else. By directing anger at them, you avoid the intimacy that would make you aware of these feelings of inadequacy.

A third way of manipulating situations that make us uncomfortable is through control. You may criticize others, telling them they aren't doing things right, or you may simply demand to know every detail of someone's activities and insist on letting her know what you think is best for her. What you are doing is keeping control of the focus in your relationships. By keeping the focus away from your own feelings of inadequacy (or fear, loneliness, and so on), you are attempting to avoid emotional pain. When you feel out of control in your inner life, it is natural to try to gain control somewhere. This control is rarely recognized by the person exercising it. Your family and friends know it well but will rarely express it. It is frightening to tell a controlling person the truth. The problem with control is that like other ways of manipulating uncomfortable situations, it makes those around you miserable and fails to solve your problem. The conditioned response is still out of your control.

Still another means of manipulating situations in order to avoid facing ourselves is through comparison. You may put yourself down by comparison with someone else. Or you may look for someone you consider inferior to yourself and pretend to feel adequate by comparison. Neither method is effective at removing the pain of isolation and inadequacy. Do you compare your marriage unfavorably to your friends' marriages? Do you avoid some social events because you feel less important (intelligent, good-looking, and so on) than the people who will be there? To compare your success with that of your peers is natural and healthy. What is not healthy is to escape from life by always seeing yourself as below (or above) another class of people.

Each of these methods allows you to manipulate the situation and ignore the emotion it makes you feel. But inside, you are still experiencing the emotion, and you will still react with depression.

You might try to look at this method of avoidance in a nonjudgmental way: instead of justifying or rationalizing your behavior, try stepping back and observing what you are doing. Is there a consistency in your pattern of avoidance? For example, do you feel fine most of the time but get nervous and develop a headache when you are asked to go out socially? If so, there is a pattern. Recognizing the pattern is important to understanding avoidance.

Step Four: Putting It All Together

In Step One, I described ways to identify your conditioned responses — even before you discover what triggers them. You focused on your habitual behavior and that of your family. In Step Two, I asked you to get in touch with the emotions that you suppress and that become the triggers for your depression. The process of getting in touch included looking at how you avoid your feelings. In Step Three, I showed you how to recognize the situations that create a depressive reaction. Your emotions do not exist in a vacuum; they are a part of how you relate to other human beings in various situations. By looking carefully at all the ways you avoid situations that make you uncomfortable, you can learn to recognize the situations that cause you to feel depressed.

Identifying your triggers and conditioned responses is a lifelong process. After you learn to recognize one set of triggers and behaviors and make changes in it, you discover another. This may sound frustrating, but it can actually be exciting. You will learn to like yourself much, much more as you take more control of your life.

How to develop positive self-control? We must learn to keep our "bell" from ringing. This includes balancing our brain chemistry so that we see things accurately. The plan that follows will help you with that. Second, we learn what our bell is, essentially following the first four steps. Next, we begin to change our situations to have control of them while we develop a reprogramming of our thoughts. For example, if I believe that what I say isn't important and I shouldn't speak in public, I might begin by sharing an idea with a small group of close friends who will ask me more about it. I will begin to learn how to present myself, and I might be encouraged about what I have to say. Next, I might present the information to a small group of individuals, perhaps my peers or colleagues. Gradually, my belief system will change to allow me to speak to thousands if I choose to. The key is to control the situation so you don't reinforce the negative emotions that began the cycle.

Problems don't just go away. You solve problems by confronting them. Please do not try to avoid what you feel, even if you need to avoid a specific situation. Your first goal is to gain self-confidence. As you learn to do that, you will gradually move out of your down moods. Your immediate goal is this: you will not allow emotions to trigger conditioned responses. Here are a few helpful suggestions for implementing Step Four.

1. Begin with self-affirmations. Focus on who you are. Tell yourself that you are worthwhile, lovable, and a creation of God.

2. Measure yourself realistically against the average. Let this give you the courage to continue to change.

3. Focus on your strengths. See what you are, not focusing on what you are not.

4. Ask for and accept compliments from your support person. Listen to others when they praise your efforts. (Don't fall into the old trap of believing they are not sincere.)

5. Carefully plan your social events. (Social events can place you in jeopardy by causing your emotions to trigger a response.) You may be uncomfortable enough initially that you will need to avoid an event or situation altogether. This is fine as long as you don't also avoid your emotions—and as long as you confront the situation again after you've gained more confidence.

6. Use the following suggestions to help yourself in social events.

   - Set a time limit for being at a social event. (If you feel comfortable, you can extend your deadline.)

   - Have an excuse ready ahead of time that will allow you to leave when you need to.

   - Explain to your spouse or support person in what way the situation is uncomfortable for you.

   - Take your spouse or support person along. They can help you combat your fears as they arise.

Finally, begin the program that follows now. This program will help you achieve confidence and accurate perceptions because your brain will be in balance. This balance will give you control over your behaviors and priorities. Then move forward boldly and with new hope. Remember, changing is frightening, but it can be rewarding. With a balanced brain and an understanding of your trigger situations, you will begin to develop new and more positive patterns. As you feel better about yourself, you will be able to change those things you never thought you could. Remember you can only change when you feel secure and confident.

Part 2   Programs
for Healing
Depression

Chapter 7

Tools That Heal

I n this chapter, I'm going to provide you with the basic tools for changing your brain chemistry and overcoming depression. How much of any one specific tool you will use will depend on whether you are a Satiation type or an Arousal type. Chapter Eight provides a complete program for overcoming Satiation depression; Chapter Nine provides the program for Arousal depression. But before we look at the individual programs, you need to know the effects of individual foods, activities, and behaviors on brain chemistry; then you can use each tool appropriately as you follow the program that best suits your needs.

What follows are dozens of powerful individual tools for changing brain chemistry and relieving depression. They are found within diet and exercise; the arts, including music, literature, theater, and films; the use of your own creative expression, such as writing, drawing, painting, and sculpture; and the enjoyment of various forms of entertainment.

Let's begin with diet.

Diet

As I have stated throughout this book, food is one of the most powerful tools for changing brain chemistry. As any lover of chocolate, sugar, or coffee will tell you, a wide variety of foods dramatically alter mood and brain function within minutes. Though most of us do not realize it, some foods have more subtle short-term effects but profound effects over the longer term. Other foods have an immediate impact on brain chemistry but tend to have the reverse effect over time. As a general rule, the greater the short-term effect of a food, behavior, or drug, the more likely that food or behavior is to then boomerang later in the opposite direction. For example, coffee speeds up neurotransmission and increases the efficiency with which the brain functions. Initially, coffee elevates mood and provides a short burst of euphoria and well-being. Several hours after the coffee is consumed, however, it causes an increase in anxiety and in nervous and muscle tension; it makes many people irritable. All caffeinated foods and beverages have similar effects, though the more caffeine a food or beverage has, the more pronounced this boomerang effect will be. Sugar is another good example. On consumption, sugar raises blood glucose levels, provides a short burst of energy, and enhances mood by significantly increasing serotonin levels in a matter of minutes. However, because sugar in the bloodstream is burned rapidly and quickly depleted, serotonin levels tend to fall just as rapidly, leaving the person with low blood sugar and low brain levels of serotonin. Another good example of this boomerang effect is alcohol, which boosts serotonin temporarily but in fact is a long-term depressant. As we saw earlier, cocaine causes a dramatic increase in norepinephrine and dopamine, but it leaves a person depleted of these neurotransmitters in the long run.

Conversely, foods that have a more balanced effect in the short term can actually cause more profound long-term effects. Take whole grains, for example. Brown rice, barley, wheat, oats, and millet boost serotonin levels in a matter of minutes. In the short run, however, this effect is more subtle than that of refined carbohydrates such as sugar.

This is because whole grains require long-term digestion and secrete their sugars into the bloodstream gradually, thus providing long-term energy and increased serotonin levels over longer periods of time. By consistently eating whole grains, we can increase and sustain higher serotonin levels; this means we can improve our baseline serotonin.

As for norepinephrine and dopamine boosters, protein-rich foods provide rapid elevations in these gas-pedal brain chemicals. So, too, do coffee, tea, and other caffeinated beverages. Because many protein-rich foods are also high in fat, I recommend that you choose low-fat animal foods, such as fish, poultry, and skim-milk products. Because protein is metabolized slowly, the boomerang effect is almost nonexistent. However, nonprotein dopamine and norepinephrine boosters, such as coffee, tea, and caffeinated beverages, can create a down feeling within hours. High-fat foods decrease oxygen to the brain and increase cholesterol, so they should be avoided.

The following subsections provide detailed lists of the foods and beverages that will boost serotonin, dopamine, and norepinephrine.

Serotonin Boosters

The best serotonin boosters in the food supply are unrefined carbohydrate-rich foods. I've listed some of the most effective here.

WHOLE GRAINS

Whole grains are essentially preserved as they are produced in nature, meaning that they have not been stripped of their fiber, germ, and nutrition in the factory. There are a multitude of whole grains. Among the most common are brown rice; sweet brown rice; wild rice (technically a grass but it can be used as a whole-grain product); barley; whole-wheat berries, whole-wheat bulgur, tabbouleh, couscous (also called semolina, it's possible to find whole-wheat couscous), and Wheatena cereal; whole oats, steel-cut oats, and rolled oats; millet; whole corn, corn on the cob, and cornmeal (also known as polenta); amaranth; teff; and quinoa.

WHOLE-GRAIN FLOUR PRODUCTS

A wide variety of whole-grain flour products exist that still contain much of their whole-grain nutrition and fiber. Once the grain is cracked to produce the flour, the food does begin to decay and lose some of its nutrition. That's why it's important to buy whole-grain breads and other flour products when they are as fresh as possible.

Whole grains that have been milled into flour are broken into tiny bits that are rapidly absorbed into the bloodstream by the small intestine. This causes an equally rapid increase in serotonin levels.

Such flour products include whole-grain breads, such as whole wheat, rye, and multiple-grain breads; pastas; chapatis; tortillas; tacos; cereals; whole-grain pasta, cereals, and other flour products, such as bagels and muffins.

SQUASH AND PUMPKIN

Squash and pumpkin are rich in carbohydrates and therefore are good serotonin boosters. They are easy to prepare by baking, boiling, or steaming. Squashes include acorn squash, butternut, buttercup, hakkaido pumpkin, Hubbard squash, pumpkin, yellow squash (also known as summer squash), and zucchini.

ROOT VEGETABLES

Rich sources of complex carbohydrates, fiber, and many important vitamins and minerals, root vegetables are also delicious serotonin boosters. They include potatoes, sweet potatoes, yams, carrots, onions, rutabagas, turnips, celery, red radish, burdock, daikon radish, and lotus root.

SNACKS AND DESSERTS

Whole-grain snacks and desserts that are rich in carbohydrates will boost serotonin levels rapidly. Virtually all of the snacks and desserts listed here can be purchased at many groceries and at natural and health food stores.

Try whole-grain cookies sweetened with apple juice, barley malt, rice syrup, or maple syrup; cakes or pastries made with whole-grain flours and sweetened with fruit juice, rice syrup, barley malt, or other natural sweeteners; whole-grain crackers; boxed cereals served with apple juice instead of milk; rice cakes with jam or rice syrup; candies made from fruit juice and other natural ingredients; popcorn; raisin breads; and corn chips made from organically grown corn and vegetable oils, such as pinta, or tortilla chips.

BEVERAGES
Fruit juice is a serotonin booster and very healthful when consumed in moderate amounts. Many varieties do contain simple sugars, however, which can adversely affect blood sugar, especially for sensitive people.

The Effects of Vegetables and Fruits on Brain Chemistry

GREEN, YELLOW, AND LEAFY VEGETABLES
Green, yellow, and leafy vegetables have a neutral effect on brain chemistry, at least in the short run, because the amount of carbohydrates in these vegetables is small and is bound up in fiber, so it takes longer to affect serotonin levels. With low carbohydrate levels, the vegetables do not boost tryptophan and serotonin as rapidly. Also, vegetables tend to be eaten with a protein-rich food, such as fish, chicken, or meat. The animal food is so rich in protein and the amino acid tyrosine that it overwhelms the effects that the small carbohydrate levels in the vegetables might have. When tryptophan and tyrosine are in the bloodstream at the same time, tyrosine gets into the brain first and converts to dopamine and norepinephrine. Therefore, the immediate effect is from the tyrosine, which overwhelms the effects of the tryptophan. Once a protein-rich food is digested and utilized, however, the remaining carbohydrate in the vegetables is available to the bloodstream; this means that over the long term, these vegetables produce small increases in serotonin levels.

Nevertheless, vegetables are among the richest sources of vitamins, minerals, and fiber in the food supply. They are especially abundant in immune-boosting and cancer-fighting nutrients, such as beta-carotene, vitamin C, and such proven cancer fighters as indoles, flavonoids, and phytochemicals.

Therefore, I urge you to eat a wide variety of fresh vegetables, including those listed here: artichokes, asparagus, bamboo shoots, beet greens, beets, broccoli, brussels sprouts, cabbage, Chinese cabbage, collard greens, cucumber, dandelion greens, dandelion root, endive, escarole, green peas, kale, kohlrabi, leeks, lettuce (preferably dark green lettuce), mushrooms (a wide variety), mustard greens, okra, scallion, sprouts, string beans, Swiss chard, and watercress.

Among the most nutritious vegetables are broccoli, cabbage, collard greens, mustard greens, and watercress.

FRUIT

Fruit has a neutral effect initially on brain chemistry because fructose, the sugar in fruit, must be converted into glucose by the small intestine in order for it to boost serotonin. This is an extremely time-consuming process that usually takes too long to have any noticeable effect on brain chemistry. Like vegetables, however, fruits such as apples, oranges, kiwis, pears, and bananas are loaded with immune boosters, fiber, and cancer-fighting nutrients.

Dopamine and Norepinephrine Boosters

FISH AND SEAFOOD

The healthiest high-protein, dopamine-and-norepinephrine-booster in the food supply is fish, simply because it is loaded with protein but low in fat. Three ounces of fish will boost your norepinephrine and dopamine levels in less than thirty minutes.

The low-fat fish that I recommend include cod, haddock, flounder, salmon, scrod, snapper, swordfish, trout, tuna, sea bass, bass, shrimp, scallops, lobster (shrimp, scallops, and lobster have low to moderate amounts of cholesterol but are generally low in fat), tuna fish (canned and preferably packed in water to avoid the oil, which is fat), sardines (canned and packed in water to avoid the fat), pickled herring, and anchovies.

CHICKEN AND TURKEY

Chicken is rich in protein; the white meat is also relatively low in fat. Avoid eating the skin of the chicken, where most of the fat is located.

For many years, people thought of turkey as a serotonin booster because it is rich in tryptophan, the precursor of serotonin. Unfortunately, turkey is far richer in protein and a wide variety of amino acids, including tyrosine, the precursor to dopamine and norepinephrine. These other amino acids compete with tryptophan to get onto the transport system that allows nutrients to pass through the blood-brain barrier. In the process, many different amino acids get onto the transport system—especially tyrosine—while only small amounts of tryptophan do. The net effect of turkey consumption, therefore, is to boost norepinephrine and dopamine.

THE PROTEIN AND FAT CONTENT OF ANIMAL FOODS

Many foods are rich in protein but even richer in fat. Protein will increase norepinephrine and dopamine, speeding up neurotransmission and increasing alertness, aggression, and arousal. In many ways, fat does just the opposite because it reduces circulation, or blood flow, especially to the brain and heart. Dietary fat and cholesterol, of course, are the leading causes of atherosclerosis, or cholesterol plaques that clog the arteries to the brain, heart, and other organs. Cholesterol plaques prevent oxygen-rich blood from getting to these and other organs, causing the organs to function at far below their optimal efficiency. Eventually, the organs suffocate, causing all or part of the organ to die. A stroke occurs when part of the brain dies; a heart attack happens when part of the heart dies.

Long before such life-threatening events occur, however, these plaques prevent the brain from getting adequate oxygen, which means that your thinking becomes dull, sluggish, and weak. Your memory may also become poor. Your speech patterns may be affected. All of this is very disturbing to the sufferer. Many people with these symptoms claim that they are simply tired, while others wonder if they are getting on in years. In fact, this diet of large quantities of fat, which leads to atherosclerosis, is precisely the underlying cause of much senility. Fortunately, many people can regain the sharpness of their mind simply by increasing the amount of oxygen flowing to the brain. You can do this by reducing the amount of fat and cholesterol in your diet. Cholesterol is only found in animal foods. All vegetable foods are free of cholesterol. Fat varies according to the food in question, so I have provided a chart that lists the fat and protein content of specific animal foods.

In general, dairy products such as milk and cheeses get approximately 25 percent of their calories from protein, 31 to 50 percent from fat, and approximately 25 percent from carbohydrates. Because dairy products are created by nature to provide nutrients for newborn cows or goats, they contain significant amounts of carbohydrates. Whole milk, for example, derives about 30 percent of its calories from carbohydrates, while skim milk derives approximately 40 percent of its calories from carbohydrates. Because milk products contain both protein and carbohydrates, their impact on brain chemistry is mixed. They also contain significant amounts of fat. The net effect of this combination of fat and carbohydrates is to make the brain sluggish.

BEANS, LEGUMES, AND BEAN PRODUCTS

Rich in protein, beans are healthful boosters of both dopamine and norepinephrine. Beans are also rich in phytoestrogens, chemicals that help prevent cancer.

There are a wide variety of beans, including adzuki beans, black-eyed peas, chickpeas, kidney beans, lima beans, lentils, navy beans, pinto beans, and soybeans (including yellow and black soybeans). There are also several very healthful and protein-rich bean products, such as tofu, tempeh, and natto. Tofu is widely available in most supermarkets and natural foods stores. Tempeh is a fermented bean product, much like cheese, that can be fried as a patty, like a hamburger, or placed in soups. Natto is a fermented soybean condiment often used in Asia on rice and other grains.

BEVERAGES

Caffeine, as mentioned before, is a short-term booster of dopamine and norepinephrine. I have provided a chart that shows the

Percent of Calories Derived from Protein and Fat

		PROTEIN	FAT

Red Meat

Red meat includes beef, lamb, veal, venison, pork, and all processed meats (such as frank-furters and sausage). Red meats are rich in protein, as well as in fat. (They often contain high levels of steroids, antibiotics, and other chemicals that may have harmful side effects, including on brain chemistry.)

		PROTEIN	FAT
BEEF	Boneless chuck, lean (with fat removed)	32%	68%
	Ground beef (hamburger)	34%	65%
	Corned beef	25%	74%
	T-bone steak (broiled)	16%	82%
	Veal, rib roast	36%	61%
LAMB	Leg	32%	66%
	Loin or lamb chops	22%	76%
PORK	Ham	21%	78%
	Pork chops, with bone	23%	75%
	Spareribs	16%	83%

Cheese

		PROTEIN	FAT
	Cottage cheese	51%	36%
	Cottage cheese (low fat)	79%	3%

Poultry

		PROTEIN	FAT
CHICKEN	White meat without skin (much of the fat in chicken is located in the skin)	76%	18%
	Dark meat without skin	64%	32%
	Fried chicken (flesh giblets)	49%	43%
EGGS	Whole	33%	65%
	Whites	85%	7%
TURKEY	Roasted	41%	56%

Fish and Seafood

	PROTEIN	FAT
Cod	89%	8%
Flounder (baked with butter or margarine; far less fat if broiled)	59%	37%
Mackerel	37%	60%
Sturgeon	63%	32%
Tuna (canned in oil)	34%	64%
Tuna (canned in water)	44%	56%
Lobster	79%	14%
Shrimp (steamed)	84%	8%
Scallops (steamed)	83%	11%

caffeine content of a variety of beverages. Here are a few additional notes on beverages.

Coffee. Coffee is an instantaneous accelerator, speeding up neurotransmission and increasing gas-pedal brain chemicals, as well as elevating endorphins. A cup of coffee contains anywhere from one hundred to two hundred milligrams of caffeine, depending on how it is brewed. In general, perked coffee has the greatest amount of caffeine, drip has less, and instant has the least. Decaffeinated coffee has a few milligrams of caffeine in it. Try to limit your coffee consumption to two cups per day, if you choose to drink it at all, because some research suggests that high doses of coffee may be linked to fibrocystic breast disease and bladder cancer.

Black tea. On average, a cup of tea contains about forty-five to one hundred milligrams of caffeine. The longer the tea is brewed, the greater the amount of caffeine it has. Tea is also rich in antioxidants and other immune-boosting and cancer-fighting nutrients.

Green tea. The average cup contains about forty-five milligrams of caffeine. Green tea usually has less caffeine than black tea. Green tea is also rich in antioxidants and has been shown to fight cancer.

Milk. As mentioned before, milk contains both protein and carbohydrates, which means that it will increase levels of both norepinephrine and serotonin. If you drink milk, be sure to use only skim or low-fat milk to avoid the fat. Another option is to use soy or rice milk.

Water. Water has a neutral effect on brain chemistry, but it's still the substance that makes up most of the human body and the drink we need the most. Since it is part of every cell and is used for transport and removal of wastes, it is important to have enough to be able to remove toxins. When we don't drink enough water, the concentration of waste products goes up, which can be harmful.

SNACKS

Seeds. Sunflower, pumpkin, and sesame seeds are dopamine and norepinephrine boosters.

Nuts. Almonds, cashews, walnuts, Brazil nuts, and others also boost dopamine and norepinephrine levels.

Caffeine Content of Beverages and Foods

Chocolate, 1 ounce (milk chocolate)	6 milligrams
Coffee, percolated	110–170 milligrams/cup (depending on brewing time)
Coffee, drip	110–150 milligrams/cup (depending on brewing time)
Coffee, instant	120 milligrams/cup
Coffee, decaffeinated	3 to 4.5 milligrams/cup
Dr. Pepper	61 milligrams/12 ounces
Coca-Cola	42 milligrams/12 ounces
Pepsi-Cola	35 milligrams/12 ounces
Diet Pepsi	34 milligrams/12 ounces
Tea, black	45–100 milligrams (depending on brewing time)

Exercise

We usually think of exercise as something that will improve our cardiovascular health, as does aerobic exercise, or increase our strength and the size of our muscles, as does weight or resistance training. But exercise is actually another important tool in changing brain chemistry and thus healing depression.

Vigorous Exercise

All vigorous exercise—such as aerobics or weight training—increases dopamine and norepinephrine while we are engaged in that activity. During the exercise, our bodies are utilizing both of these gas-pedal chemicals in order to support muscle activity, heart rate, respiration, and nerve function. Once the exercise is over, however, the higher levels of dopamine and norepinephrine have been burned off, while serotonin levels increase. This elevation in serotonin is associated with feelings of well-being and satisfaction with oneself for having exercised. The body offers a biochemical reward for exercise to encourage us to keep doing it.

This is not where things stop, however. The drop in norepinephrine and dopamine is temporary. Both of these chemicals tend to increase gradually over the next few days, making us restless and anxious and giving rise to the need to exercise again. We exercise again, then experience a sense of well-being and satisfaction with ourselves, and start the cycle all over. This cycle is further evidence of the body's wisdom, for in encouraging us to exercise, it is of course promoting health, longevity—and a balanced brain chemistry.

Research has shown that exercise reduces both depression and anxiety. After only twenty minutes of running, the brain secretes elevated levels of beta endorphins, which are morphinelike compounds that create the "natural high" that runners frequently talk about. A study published in the scientific journal *Obesity* (5:557, 1981) found that only twenty minutes of running per day relieves depression. Today we amend that recommendation to include up to four days a week for twenty minutes per day.

Another study examining the effects of regular exercise on patients in a psychiatric hospital found that exercise significantly decreased depression and anxiety and increased a sense of accomplishment and well-being.

Finally, all competitive sports or games increase levels of norepinephrine and dopamine and will keep them elevated, especially if you become personally invested in the outcome of the game. If you do become especially attached to winning but you lose, you will suffer the effects of low serotonin and elevated norepinephrine long after the game has been played. If you win, your serotonin levels will increase, but your norepinephrine levels will also stay elevated. This means that you will be restless for some time after the game is over. These changes in brain chemistry tend to be proportional to your attachment to winning. The more personally invested you are in winning, the lower your serotonin levels will be when you lose and the higher they will be when you win. When we are in a competitive state we release dopamine and norepinephrine. The exercise may not be enough to burn up this increase. Therefore, noncompetitive, vigorous exercise is the best way to decrease norepinephrine and dopamine.

Stretching and Gentle Exercise

Gentle exercise, such as stretching, strolling, ballroom dancing, or yoga, mildly increases dopamine and norepinephrine but significantly boosts serotonin levels. These exercises are wonderful ways to warm up and cool down after vigorous exercise. They are also especially helpful at balancing brain chemistry on those days when you do not exercise vigorously.

People who want to boost serotonin without elevating dopamine and norepinephrine should adopt a program that includes gentle stretching, strolling, or low-impact aerobics. These exercises are especially good when done in a natural setting, such as in a forest or by the ocean.

The following lists provide specific examples of exercises that have a positive effect on brain chemistry.

Serotonin Boosters

- Walking and strolling on a flat surface
- Walking in nature (through a forest, along the beach, in a park)
- Riding a bicycle on a flat surface with low exertion
- Stretching
- Low-impact aerobics
- Gentle weight lifting, using low weights
- Ballroom dancing

Exercises That Lower Dopamine and Norepinephrine (Temporarily) and Boost Serotonin

- Aerobic dancing
- Cross-country skiing
- Jogging
- Strenuous bicycling

- Riding a stationary bicycle
- Using the Stairmaster
- Using a rowing machine
- Using the Nautilus machines
- Walking or running on a treadmill
- Hiking, especially uphill
- Swimming
- Doing water aerobics
- Strenuous weight lifting
- Playing basketball (as long as you are not so competitive that your self-esteem depends on the outcome of the game)
- Playing tennis (as long as you are not overly competitive)
- Playing racquetball (as long as you are not overly competitive)
- Fast or highly rhythmic dancing, such as swing dancing, contra dancing, rumba, tango, and dancing to rock and roll

Exercises That Boost Dopamine and Norepinephrine

All competitive sports and any physical activity in which you are invested in winning will raise dopamine and norepinephrine and burn them off somewhat, but they may keep both brain chemicals elevated if you take the competition too seriously. These activities include:

- Basketball
- Tennis
- Racquetball
- Wrestling
- Competitive swimming
- Competitive weight lifting
- Competitive track events (sprints, long-distance running, hurdles, javelin, shot put, and others)

Nature: Shifting Moods, Rising Tides

In general, being in nature—such as in a forest, in the desert, at the beach, or near the ocean—is a serotonin booster. If you combine a gentle exercise such as walking with such settings, their effects on serotonin are even more pronounced. Thus, walking in the woods, on the beach, or in the desert (especially at night when the desert is cooler) can have a pronounced effect on serotonin levels, elevating your mood and leaving you feeling relaxed.

Serotonin Boosters in Nature

- Canoeing, rafting, and boating, especially on a gentle river or calm lake or ocean
- Walking in a park or forest
- Sitting near a body of water or in a boat on the water
- Floating or gentle swimming, especially in a calm lake or pool

Norepinephrine and Dopamine Boosters

In contrast, white-water rafting, being at sea during a storm, hiking in the woods during high winds or a thunderstorm (especially if there's lightning), or trekking through the tundra or polar regions will trigger our survival mechanisms and increase norepinephrine and dopamine. There are many safe and enjoyable ways to be in nature and elevate norepinephrine and dopamine. I've listed some of the most popular here.

- Boating and rafting, especially on a fast river (Do not push yourself beyond your knowledge, skill, or personal limits. Use a guide where necessary or enjoy a gentler river; this will still increase your gas-pedal chemicals.)
- Speedboating

- Kayaking, especially on a fast river
- Skulling, especially in competition
- Rowing, especially when it becomes vigorous
- Mountain climbing (Again, stay within your skill, knowledge, and physical limits.)
- Running and brisk walking in nature
- Exploring a large and unfamiliar forest, especially one in which a lot of wildlife lives (You should go exploring with experienced people who are familiar with that forest.)
- Bungee jumping
- Skydiving
- Hang gliding
- Rock rapelling
- Swimming, especially in the ocean

As a general rule, nature in its gentler phases boosts serotonin. Sunshine, clear skies, and a mild wind are all recognized as serotonin boosting. Rain and dark winter weather, on the other hand, cause a decline in serotonin. Interestingly, many people find falling snow very calming and supportive. It creates images of coziness and warm fires, both of which increase serotonin.

Whenever nature is aroused and violent, it boosts norepinephrine and dopamine. Wind, hard rain, hail, mud slides, hurricanes, tornadoes, earthquakes, volcanoes—you get the picture—are definitely norepinephrine and dopamine producing.

Music: Gentle Ways to Change Brain Chemistry and Mood

Music is one of the most powerful tools for changing brain chemistry. It alters our chemistry instantly, with no known negative side effects. If chosen well, music can be medicine for the mind and soul.

Virtually all the great composers have created music that alternately boosted serotonin and increased norepinephrine and dopamine. Compare the slow movement of a Beethoven symphony to a fast movement, for example. But almost every composer also created certain pieces that maintain a particular spirit and mood. This means that we can use individual pieces of great music to change our brain chemistries in a matter of minutes, if not seconds.

In order to help you explore the effects of music on brain chemistry, I offer here a short list of composers and artists, along with examples of their music that boost either serotonin or norepinephrine. Remember that this is just a sampling; it would be impossible within the scope of this book to provide a comprehensive list of pieces or composers! I encourage you to explore the realm of music and its effects on brain chemistry. It's a great way to maintain a certain atmosphere in your life—either calming, soothing, and serotonin boosting, or exciting, inspiring, and norepinephrine boosting.

Please remember that this list is rather subjective. This is a general list that may not fit you; you will need to tailor it for your own use.

Serotonin Boosters

CLASSICAL COMPOSERS

Bach: especially the *Brandenburg Concertos* and "Jesu, Joy of Man's Desiring"

Beethoven: "Ode to Joy" (the choral movement from his Ninth Symphony)

Chopin: especially his Preludes. Roy Eaton's *The Meditative Chopin* combines a variety of serotonin-boosting pieces from Chopin for piano.

Handel: especially *Water Music*

Mozart: Allegro from Sonata Facile no. 16; Adagio from Clarinet Concerto; Andante from Piano Concerto no. 21; Overture from *The Magic Flute*; many others

Pachelbel: Canon. The Canon is now being produced with ocean sounds in the background—very calming, soothing, and serotonin boosting.

~ Vivaldi: especially *The Four Seasons*, a major serotonin booster

FOLK MUSIC

Virtually all folk music is serotonin boosting. Choose any of the old favorites that most appeal to you.

JAZZ AND RHYTHM AND BLUES

Rhythm and blues can be pretty depressing, especially if you're already depressed. Don't get me wrong—this genre offers a lot of great music, but most of the lyrics focus on life's travails. Many people find such music highly cathartic, emotional, and healing, but others can be brought even lower by the deep suffering that the music often expresses. Therefore, I recommend exercising some caution in this category, at least until you feel ready to deal with your own deep emotional pain.

Jazz, on the other hand, can be incredibly uplifting and joyful. It can be melodic and soothing (thus a serotonin booster) or exciting and arousing (a norepinephrine booster). Choose the pieces you especially enjoy for their desired effects.

ROCK AND ROLL

Most rock and roll is norepinephrine and dopamine boosting. However, rock is often hard to classify. Even hard rock bands produce serotonin-boosting songs from time to time, such as Guns and Roses' *November Rain*. Also, some people think of the Beatles and Simon and Garfunkle, for example, as rock artists, though a great many of the Beatles' songs are serotonin boosters (*I Will; Here, There, and Everywhere; Something; Michele;* and many others), just as are most of Simon and Garfunkle's music (*Bridge over Troubled Water* is the classic example). There are many rock artists who produce softer serotonin-boosting music. Once you get the hang of classifying music according to its effects on brain chemistry, you'll be able to go through your musical library and choose accordingly.

MUSICAL THEATER

The music of musical theater is generally upbeat and inspiring. Many of the stories have a happy ending, and this boosts serotonin, too. Of course, there are exceptions, such as Leonard Bernstein's *West Side Story* and Andrew Lloyd Webber's *Miss Saigon*—musicals that offer perhaps more catharsis than uplift. The following list includes the names of some classic serotonin-boosting musicals.

Cole Porter: *Anything Goes* and others

Oscar Hammerstein and Richard Rogers: *Oklahoma, The Sound of Music, Carousel, South Pacific*, and many others

Frank Loesser: *Guys and Dolls* and others

Andrew Lloyd Webber: *Cats, Phantom of the Opera*, and others

Stephen Sondheim: *A Little Night Music* and many others

Marvin Hamlish: *A Chorus Line*

Alan Jay Lerner and Frederick Loewe: *My Fair Lady*

Norepinephrine and Dopamine Boosters

CLASSICAL COMPOSERS

Beethoven: most of the music from the Fifth and Ninth Symphonies is arousing and will boost dopamine and norepinephrine

Kabalevsky: "Gallop" from Opus 39, no. 18

Mozart: Overture from *The Marriage of Figaro*; Menuetto from *A Little Night Music*; Serenade no. 13

Tchaikovsky: most of *The Nutcracker* is arousing, as is much of Tchaikovsky's music

ROCK AND ROLL

Most of modern rock and roll is arousing and consequently will boost norepinephrine and dopamine. There are endless choices to suit your tastes. Bruce Springstein's album *Born to Run* is a classic norepinephrine and dopamine booster.

Writing and the Power of Confession

In general, writing in a journal is a powerful serotonin booster. On the other hand, it can also elevate norepinephrine and dopamine when you write about life events that have been especially painful or terrifying. Writing about such events can be a safe way to confront old wounds that you may have been avoiding. Research has shown that writing about such events and confronting them honestly can restore psychic equilibrium and overcome depression.

In the early 1980s, James W. Pennebaker, a professor of psychology at Southern Methodist University in Dallas, Texas, experienced a deep depression that he could not shake. He became introverted, isolated himself, stopped eating, and refused to seek counseling. He had just married, and the sudden change in his life brought to the surface many deep issues that he had not dealt with before. These lingering issues, he discovered, had brought on his depression.

As a way of exploring his own pain, he began to write about his life in a private journal. He began with his earliest experiences and wrote up to the present time. He was looking for the source of his pain. What he found in the act of writing—especially in writing about the traumatic events that had occurred in his life—was a cure for his depression.

In his book, *Opening Up: The Healing Power of Confiding in Others* (Avon, 1991), Pennebaker describes the powerful effect that writing had on his inner state. "For the first time in years—perhaps ever—I had a sense of meaning and direction. I fundamentally understood my deep love for my wife and the degree to which I needed her. It wasn't until eight years later that I looked back on that period in an attempt to understand why writing had been so helpful."

In the late 1980s and early 1990s, Pennebaker teamed up with immunologist Ronald Glaser and psychologist Janice Kiecolt-Glaser to study the effects of writing about deeply painful events on a person's immune system and psychological health. He devised what became known as "the Pennebaker method." This method asked participants in the study to write for four days in a row for at least twenty minutes per day about the most traumatic and painful event in their lives. Since Pennebaker was a professor at a large institution, he could administer his method to large groups of students.

The study participants had to write about a specific traumatic event in their lives, an event that they had never talked about with anyone, or an event that contained information that the participant had never shared before. Pennebaker stressed that it was especially important that the student write about the pain, anger, remorse, and guilt he or she may have felt about the event. As Pennebaker points out, many of these students had suffered deeply painful and even traumatic events, including sexual abuse. After the student completed his or her four days of journal writing, he or she turned the journal in to Pennebaker.

Glaser and Kiecolt-Glaser ran a series of psychological and immunological tests on each student before and after he or she did the journal writing. In this way, they were able to determine what, if any, effect the journal writing had on the students' physical and psychological condition.

What the scientists found was remarkable. Not only did the journal writing boost the immune responses of the students but it also improved their psychological health. The scientists found that both immune and psychological conditions were significantly better after the writing exercises than before. The number and aggressiveness of T-cells—cells that organize an immune response to a disease-causing agent—had increased significantly in the students who did the four days of confessional writing as compared to their matched controls who did not do the writing. Moreover, the study group had fewer visits to the health clinic than the control group. The immune response was especially strong in the students who confided feelings and experiences that they had never talked about or shared with anyone. These people, whom Pennebaker termed "high disclosers," had the most remarkable improvement in T-cell response and psychological health, as evidenced by decreased depression, anxiety, and stress.

Further research by Pennebaker revealed why the writing had such a powerful effect on both mental and physical health. He argued that the mechanism by which we keep feelings hidden—a mechanism he refers to as psychological inhibition—requires tremendous amounts of psychic and physical energy. As he describes it, inhibition is demanding work, especially when a very painful trauma must be kept secret. Such inhibition frequently brings on physical symptoms, such as elevations in blood pressure, heart rate, breathing, skin temperature, and perspiration levels. As Pennebaker found in his own life and in the lives of his study participants, inhibition can also be the basis for depression.

Pennebaker spoke with FBI agents who conduct polygraph (lie detector) tests on suspected criminals, and their experiences corroborated his study. During a polygraph test, the suspect undergoes physical stress that creates electrical signals, which the polygraph machine interprets to determine if the person is telling the truth or lying. From working with the FBI agents, Pennebaker learned that when a suspect confesses his crime, his physical symptoms of inhibition—among which are muscle tension, exaggerated electrical responses, elevated heart and respiratory rate—all disappear. In other words, confession has a dramatic impact on our psychological and physical conditions.

Pennebaker also found that when criminals confess during polygraph tests, they often feel bonded to their confessors; many send them Christmas cards and letters later, thanking them for their help. The confession, in effect, has restored balance to the psychological and physical condition of the suspect. With this restoration of balance come feelings of peace, tranquillity, and resolution, as well as better health.

The same phenomenon occurs in people who use the Pennebaker method. During the first two days of writing, people tend to experience negative emotions, such as anger, sadness, anxiety, and grief. On the third or fourth day, however, they begin to experience feelings of relief, insight, and resolution, suggesting that they have released the inhibiting energy and integrated the traumatic events into their consciousness.

Pennebaker points out that one does not necessarily have to *write* about the event. Confessing it aloud to someone else will have the same effect.

The rules for writing such confessions are simple enough:

1. Write for twenty minutes for four consecutive days.
2. Write continuously about the most upsetting experience or trauma of your entire life.
3. Don't worry about grammar, spelling, or the structure of the piece.
4. Write your deepest thoughts and emotions regarding the experience. Include all the details you can remember and any insights you gain into the event and your feelings.

I strongly encourage anyone who is depressed to try this exercise. Don't limit your writing to four days, however. Concentrate on a single event and write about it for four days for at least twenty minutes per writing session. Once you have completed one round of the exercise, do it again for other painful events in your life.

The more you become intimate with yourself, the more you release these inhibiting psychic barriers. This will change your baseline by elevating your serotonin and decreasing your dopamine and norepinephrine and, in the process, help you overcome your depression.

Other artistic pursuits can have similar effects on brain chemistry, I believe. For those who are drawn to painting, drawing, or sculpture, you can also use these pursuits to heal old wounds and reestablish balance in your mind and brain chemistry. Drawing, sculpting, or painting to express your feelings or an emotion you felt during a past traumatic event can be very cathartic. When emotions that were hidden are expressed, serotonin goes up and norepinephrine and dopamine decrease.

Entertainment Tools

Different forms of entertainment can serve as tools to help balance our brain chemistry, or they can have a negative impact on our minds and moods. For many of us today, for example, television has become a drug. We use it to escape our feelings and to medicate our brains. Some shows are serotonin boosters, but most are highly arousing and therefore increase norepinephrine and dopamine. Similarly, the vast majority of films today—action, suspense, thriller, or horror movies—boost dopamine and norepinephrine. The increase in these chemicals causes tremendous tension that cannot be easily released, especially if we are sitting still while our brain chemistries are being manipulated.

Depressed people—both Satiation and Arousal types—particularly use television to help them avoid experiencing their feelings. This form of avoidance can be just as much of a drug as alcohol and marijuana.

I recommend that all depressed people avoid television and instead write in a journal, listen to music, exercise, or participate in some other activity that balances brain chemistry. If you are looking for an escape, go out to a movie; the effort of getting out of the house is mildly arousing and healthier than sitting in front of the TV.

Spiritual Practices and Religion

Most individual spiritual practices, such as prayer and meditation, and all meditative church, synagogue, and temple services boost serotonin levels. On the other hand, emotional preaching, singing, and arousing spiritual practices, such as those common in the Pentecostal faith, boost norepinephrine and dopamine.

Obviously, individual prayer, meditation, and quiet services will appeal to Satiation types, while highly arousing singing and services will appeal to Arousal types. If you are in need of increasing serotonin, you may wish to spend more time in prayer and meditation. This increase in serotonin may help to decrease greater than optimal levels of norepinephrine and dopamine. If you need to increase dopamine and norepinephrine, you may find that motivational and emotional preaching will help you.

The brain-chemistry model can be used to assess the impact of every activity on serotonin, dopamine, and norepinephrine. This chapter should give you a good idea of how to apply the model to activities not listed here. Now let's turn to the specific programs that will help heal Satiation and Arousal depression.

Chapter 8

A Program for Healing Satiation Depression

General Treatment Approach

As we described in Chapter Four, if you are suffering from Satiation depression, you have low levels of serotonin as well as low levels of norepinephrine and dopamine. Our strategy, then, should be to raise your serotonin and gently raise your norepinephrine and dopamine to give you a greater sense of personal power. We can accomplish this by following these four general guidelines:

1. Adopt the brain-chemistry model for the Satiation-depressed personality, designed to balance your brain chemistry and help you overcome your depression.

2. Develop a stronger sense of self. Start to feel your feelings; without condemning yourself, acknowledge your current sense of powerlessness, and recognize your desire for a better life. Knowing yourself is the first and most important step to being able to satisfy your deepest desires. I strongly recommend writing daily in a journal and using the Pennebaker method.

3. Open up to new possibilities and a new way of living. Know that your current brain chemistry is shaping your perceptions and limiting what you believe to be possible. With time and application of this program, your brain chemistry will change, and new possibilities will become available to you. Understand that there are more opportunities for change and a better life than you may currently be able to see. Without focusing on any of your own limitations, acknowledge that it is possible to regain your emotional strength and health. You can restore your physical vitality and develop a greater sense of personal power. This program will show you how.

4. As you adopt the program and start to feel your inner strength increase, confront your stressors more directly. Avoid the television and other Satiation activities that anesthetize you to what is really bothering you. Try to deal with life more directly and honestly.

The program outlined here consists of diet, exercise, and lifestyle factors. All of these are tools for changing brain chemistry and relieving the symptoms of depression. Most of these recommendations are designed to raise serotonin levels and maintain these higher levels over time. These alone will improve your self-esteem, well-being, confidence, and sense of personal safety. Other recommendations are designed to raise norepinephrine and dopamine gradually and gently, giving you a greater sense of personal power, authenticity, alertness, speedier neurotransmission, and more energy.

Let's begin by outlining the diet you should follow to accomplish your goals.

A Diet for the Satiation-Depressed Person

Before you start any diet program, you need to recognize that as a Satiation personality type there are certain foods that have a particularly strong impact on your emotional health.

1. *Carbohydrates.* You may be relying on sugar, alcohol, and/or refined carbohydrates, such as white-flour products, to medicate your fears, anxiety, and tension. Sugar, refined carbohydrates, and alcohol may be weakening you significantly; in all likelihood, they are contributing to your depression. Controlling these foods is essential to your recovery.

My Recommendation: Significantly reduce or eliminate all refined-flour products, all refined white sugar, and all alcohol. Substitute whole-grain flour products for white-flour foods; use more natural sugars, such as fruit juices, barley malt, rice syrup, and maple syrup for sugar; and drink nonalcoholic beer or wine, sparkling water, water, or fruit juice instead of alcohol.

2. *Protein-rich foods.* Protein increases blood levels of tyrosine, and this in turn promotes production of norepinephrine and dopamine. Protein can be utilized to give you more energy and to promote a stronger sense of self, greater alertness, assertiveness, and aggression. As long as you are not weakening yourself with refined carbohydrates and alcohol, the combination of whole-grain products and healthful amounts of protein can help make you much stronger, more confident, and more effective.

My Recommendation: Begin by eating protein-rich foods from animal sources two times a week. As you feel more comfortable with these foods and the increase in energy and assertiveness they provide, increase the frequency to three times a week. Between these protein meals, eat whole grains, whole-grain products, fresh vegetables, and fruit. This combination of foods will boost serotonin and gently increase norepinephrine and dopamine, all of which will dramatically transform your brain chemistry.

These two aspects of your diet are essential to changing your emotional condition and restoring your health. You can make the changes in the factors that you feel comfortable with, but the more you adhere to these recommendations, the more profound the effects will be on your inner state.

General Dietary Guidelines

The goal of this program is to increase serotonin as quickly as possible, while gently and gradually increasing norepinephrine and dopamine. The following general recommendations will accomplish this.

1. Eat a whole-grain food at every meal. These foods include brown rice, barley, corn, millet, oats, whole wheat, whole-wheat bread, chapatis, corn tortillas and tacos, and rye bread. Make a whole grain your first choice (refer to the lists in Chapter Seven); your second choice should be a whole-grain flour product, such as whole-wheat or seven-grain bread.

2. Snack on whole grains and foods made of whole-grain flour. Examples include rice cakes, whole-grain cookies, popcorn, whole-grain pastries, and raisin bread.

3. Eat a low-fat, protein-rich food, such as fish or the white meat of poultry, twice a week. Supplement these foods with daily helpings of vegetable-protein foods, such as beans, tofu, tempeh, soy milk, soy cheese, and others.

4. Reduce or eliminate from your diet high-fat animal products, including many forms of red meat and dairy foods. Not only do these foods harm your overall health but they will reduce serotonin levels and contribute to your depression.

5. Significantly reduce or eliminate all caffeinated beverages and foods, such as chocolate, coffee, and some teas.

A Daily Eating Plan

Whole grains. At least twice a day and preferably at every meal. These are essential to your diet to increase serotonin. These include brown rice, barley, oats, millet, and others. Boil or pressure-cook them.

Whole-grain flour products. Daily. When you do not have a whole grain at a meal, eat a whole-grain flour product to maintain your serotonin levels. Whole-grain flour foods include pastas, whole-wheat bread, rye bread, and whole-grain muffins, desserts, and snacks.

Puffed grains and cereals. When desired. These include Raisin Bran, Wheaties, Cheerios, and many others. If you would like to avoid dairy products, use soy milk or apple juice as a substitute for milk.

Green, leafy, and/or yellow vegetables. Once or twice daily. These include collard greens, kale, mustard greens, broccoli, and others.

Root vegetables. Two or three times per week. These include onion, celery, turnips, rutabagas, and others.

Fresh fruit. Daily. Dried fruits—whenever desired.

Fish. Once or twice a week. The list includes cod, scrod, flounder, halibut, salmon, and others. (All are low in fat; salmon contains omega polyunsaturated fats, which lower blood cholesterol.)

Chicken. Once a week, if desired. Remove the skin before eating.

Menu Suggestions

BREAKFAST
The following breakfast suggestions boost serotonin levels.

- Oatmeal with raisins or other fruit, or with honey or rice syrup
- Oatmeal mixed with bulgur wheat, rice, Wheatena, or other grains

- Leftover brown rice: the dinner rice can be reheated with more water to make it wetter and looser for the morning meal.
- Toast with jams (preferably those with no sugar added)
- Whole-grain muffin
- English muffin
- Hash browns
- Cereals, preferably with no added sugar: puffed rice and other puffed whole grains, Wheaties, Cheerios, Raisin Bran, and many others. If you would like to avoid dairy products, use apple juice as a substitute for milk.
- Fruit juice

Any of the following breakfast suggestions will boost dopamine and norepinephrine levels.

- Any type of fish or fish soup
- Smoked salmon (lox)
- Sliced tofu on toast, with a few drops of tamari or soy sauce or balsamic vinegar, or with grated ginger root
- Black tea
- Green tea
- Coffee

LUNCH
The following lunch suggestions will boost serotonin levels.

- A whole grain: brown rice, millet, barley, and corn are among those listed in Chapter Seven.
- A green vegetable: collard greens, kale, mustard greens, turnip greens, and broccoli are among the best.
- A root or squash or other vegetable: this can include carrots, daikon radish, or some other vegetable listed in Chapter Seven.
- A piece of fresh fruit, preferably in season
- Leftover grain from dinner

- Sandwiches composed of whole-grain bread, leafy green vegetables (such as collard greens or kale), salad, mustard, balsamic vinegar, olive oil
- Pasta
- Hash brown potatoes
- Greens and mixed vegetable salad
- Lightly steamed or sautéed vegetables
- Vegetable soup, such as minestrone
- Whole-grain burgers, with a variety of toppings, on whole-grain bread or bun: available in stores, they need only be thawed and heated in the morning before work or at lunch.
- Wide variety of whole-grain chapati sandwiches, consisting of brown rice and vegetables wrapped in chapati: widely available in natural foods stores

The following lunch suggestions will boost dopamine and norepinephrine levels.

- Tuna salad sandwich
- Chicken or turkey salad sandwich
- Fish sandwich
- Fish (any type)
- Beans
- Tofu hot dogs
- Tacos with beans
- Tortillas with beans
- Bean chili

DINNER

The following dinner suggestions will boost serotonin levels.

- A whole grain, such as brown rice, wild rice, barley, millet (pressure-cooked or boiled), tabbouleh, others; with any number of condiments: many grains can be purchased prepackaged and ready to be heated and served.

- Vegetable or grain soup
- Pasta: any one of a wide variety of noodles with marinara sauce or some other vegetable topping of your choice
- Steamed or sautéed leafy green vegetable
- Baked squash
- A root vegetable or vegetable medley that includes roots, mushrooms, and broccoli
- Salad with a variety of leafy greens, celery, carrot, cucumber

The following dinner suggestions will boost dopamine and norepinephrine.

- Broiled fish: any type in any preparation desired (avoid frying)
- Chicken, turkey
- Beans (see lunch suggestions)
- Bean burrito, taco, chapati
- Tofu and tempeh

Some General Thoughts About the Dietary Plan

In order to make the suggested dietary adjustments as easy and as comfortable as possible, I recommend that you gradually decrease foods that are rich in protein and refined carbohydrates, which are contributing significantly to your current brain-chemistry imbalance. As you decrease the amount of red meat, eggs, and other high-fat, high-protein foods that you eat, increase vegetable foods, such as whole grains, fresh vegetables, beans, and fruit. These foods will balance your neurotransmitters and restore harmony to your inner state.

COMPLEX CARBOHYDRATE SNACKS

Two hours after your largest protein meal, snack on a complex carbohydrate food, such as those listed in Chapter Seven. A rice cake, a slice of whole-wheat toast, or a couple of whole-wheat crackers may be all it takes. Don't add more calories, just replace the calories with this snack.

This snack helps keep tyrosine and tryptophan from competing to enter the brain. Two hours after you have eaten, the tyrosine is already absorbed, and the tryptophan is still in the blood. Snacking on the complex carbohydrate drives the tryptophan into the brain, thus balancing the brain chemistry.

This technique, used for a couple of weeks, will help decrease anxious feelings and "down" time in the afternoon for those sleeping at night.

WHERE WILL I GET MY PROTEIN?

Many people worry about whether they will get adequate protein if they begin to decrease the animal foods in their diet and increase whole grains, fresh vegetables, and beans. In fact, nutrition scientists point out that a completely vegetarian diet contains all the protein an adult needs to maintain optimal health.

Protein is used by the body for the creation of hormones, cell replacement and repair, and the production of body hair. In order to meet and exceed all of the body's requirements for protein, an adult must eat approximately twenty grams of protein a day, which amounts to about two-thirds of an ounce. You can get that much protein and more per day just by eating your fill of potatoes. I'm not suggesting that you eat only potatoes; the point is that as long as you eat a diet based largely on whole foods—such as whole, unrefined grains and vegetables, beans, and fruit—you cannot become deficient in protein, even if the diet is composed entirely of vegetables. All whole, unrefined vegetable foods contain complete protein. In fact, no nutritionist can create a diet made up of whole vegetable foods that is inadequate in protein, even for a child.

On the other hand, you do not need to become a vegetarian. There are plenty of animal foods listed on the diet. Fish and poultry are rich sources of protein.

You can also adjust your protein intake to suit your own needs. Keep in mind, however, that most Americans today eat far too much protein to maintain their physical and mental health. Science has demonstrated that excess protein is linked to osteoporosis, kidney disorders, and several types of cancer. The National Academy of Sciences, the office of the U.S. surgeon general, and other prestigious scientific groups have encouraged Americans to reduce their intake of protein-rich foods and especially reduce the consumption of animal protein. The reason is simple: many of the animal sources of protein are high-fat foods, especially red meats, eggs, and many dairy products. The only exceptions to this are fish and the white meat of poultry. All animal foods have cholesterol, as well.

By eating large amounts of fat and protein, you increase your risk of a whole host of degenerative diseases, including heart disease, cancer, adult-onset diabetes, and other serious disorders.

OTHER IMPORTANT CONSIDERATIONS

1. If a physician has suggested an alternative diet due to a medical condition or for any other reason, please follow that advice.

2. If you have food allergies, use alternative foods.

3. High-sodium foods may be inappropriate if you have high blood pressure or certain other medical conditions.

4. The goal of this diet is not to reduce your weight but to provide a balanced diet for your brain.

5. The body needs carbohydrates to function. Complex carbohydrates (such as whole grains, rice, potatoes, and pasta) are the most effective foods for increasing serotonin and maintaining balanced moods.

6. Eat at least three meals a day of the approved foods.

7. Avoid all alcohol and nonprescribed medications or drugs.

8. Trim all visible fat from poultry, fish, and meat.

9. Replace saturated fats with polyunsaturated fats and decrease the amount of fats consumed. To cut back on saturated fats, you can cut back on animal fats and trim excess fat from meat. It can also help to use cooking oils that are lower in saturated fats, such as

canola or safflower oil. Remember that although margarine has lower saturated fat than butter, it is still a rather high-fat food.

10. Minimize your consumption of high-cholesterol foods.

11. Avoid or minimize your consumption of processed or refined sugars.

12. Minimize the use of salt and foods high in salt content.

13. Choose fresh foods over processed foods.

14. Avoid frying or immersing foods in oil; instead, broil, steam, or bake foods as much as possible.

15. Please consult your physician if you have any questions or suffer from other medical problems.

Your Daily Exercise Plan

The goal of this exercise program is to increase your brain levels of serotonin significantly and rapidly, while making modest increases in norepinephrine and dopamine. There are two types of exercises to choose from: one group that relaxes, referred to as "R" activities, and another that excites, called "E."

A Cautionary Note Before You Begin

Before you begin any exercise or activity program, you should consult your physician to determine if you have any physical limitations or preexisting conditions that could become worse with exercise. If after you begin your exercise plan, your symptoms worsen or you feel more depressed or anxious, please discontinue the activity and consult your physician.

Research has shown that certain types of exercise and activities can have both immediate and long-term effects on brain chemistry and overall health. The program suggested here can enhance your brain chemistry when followed consistently. These suggestions are based on what I have found to be a generally safe and effective exercise program for a Satiation-depressed person. You may need to modify the program somewhat to meet your individual needs, scheduling demands, and lifestyle. When making modifications, use the guidelines outlined in Chapters Three and Seven. In general, your exercise program should increase serotonin and gradually increase norepinephrine and dopamine.

General Guidelines for Your Activity Program

There are two categories of exercise and activities that affect brain chemistry. The first type, called relaxing (designated with an R), boosts serotonin levels, while the second, called exciting (designated with an E), increases norepinephrine and dopamine when performed at least three times weekly for six to eight weeks. Prior to that, it may actually "burn up" norepinephrine and dopamine. Relaxing activities do not significantly increase your heart rate, while exciting activities tend to be aerobic or physically demanding.

For more on Satiation exercises designed to boost serotonin and Arousal exercises to increase norepinephrine, see Chapter Three.

EXAMPLES OF "R" ACTIVITIES

Stretching exercises

Walking slow on a flat surface (strolling)

Biking on a flat surface

Camping

Canoeing in calm waters

Fishing

Woodworking

See Chapter Seven for a list of more "R," or serotonin-boosting, activities.

EXAMPLES OF "E" ACTIVITIES

Running

Mountain climbing

Hunting

Weight lifting

Swimming

Hiking

Aerobics

Racquet sports

Mountain biking

Competitive sports

See Chapter Seven for a list of more "E," or norepinephrine-boosting, activities.

As you read these lists, pick out the ones you enjoy most, and consider how you can incorporate them into your schedule and lifestyle. Choose the ones you will be willing to do on a consistent basis. Next consider your present exercise schedule. How often are you doing an "R" activity? How often are you doing an "E" activity?

If you are not exercising at all now, use the first schedule here for your new exercise program. If you are already exercising, use the second.

If you are not particularly fond of exercising, follow these guidelines:

1. Perform a five-minute warm-up such as walking or stretching.

2. Perform a twenty-minute exercise from the "R" list.

3. Perform a five-minute cooldown such as walking or stretching.

DAILY SCHEDULE

Sun.	Mon.	Tue.	Wed.	Thur.	Fri.	Sat.
R	R	R	R	R	R	R

Exercise Program 1 for People Not Exercising Now

Sun.	Mon.	Tue.	Wed.	Thur.	Fri.	Sat.
R	E/R	R	E/R	R	E/R	R

Perform a five-minute warm-up (R), such as stretching and walking, before doing an arousing or demanding exercise (E). Once you have warmed up, do twenty minutes of E or R exercises, depending on which day it is. After you do an E activity, do another five minutes of R activities, such as stretching and/or walking, as a way of cooling down.

A Sample Week of Exercise

Sunday: A relaxing activity, such as walking in nature or in a park; stretching (R).

Monday: Five minutes of stretching or low-impact aerobics (R), followed by a brisk walk, jog, or bicycle ride of at least twenty minutes (E) or some competitive game, such as tennis, racquetball, or basketball (E). Followed by stretching (R).

Tuesday: Twenty minutes of stretching warm-up, low-impact aerobics, or a slow walk or stroll (R).

Wednesday: Five minutes of stretching or low-impact aerobic warm-up (R). A brisk walk, jog, or bicycle ride of at least twenty minutes (E) or a competitive game (E). Stretching cooldown (R).

Thursday: Twenty minutes of stretching, low-impact aerobics, or stroll (R).

Friday: Five minutes of stretching or low-impact aerobics (R). A brisk walk, jog, or bicycle ride of at least twenty minutes (E) or a competitive sport (E). Stretching as a cooldown (R).

Saturday: Twenty minutes of stretching, strolling, fishing, canoeing, or some other relaxing activity (R).

Exercise Program 2 for People Who Exercise Now

Sun.	Mon.	Tue.	Wed.	Thur.	Fri.	Sat.
R	E/R	E/R	E/R	E/R	R or E/R	R

Perform a five-minute warm-up (R), such as stretching and walking, before doing an arousing or demanding exercise (E). Once you have warmed up, do twenty minutes of E or R exercises, depending on the day in question, and then another five minutes of cooldown activities (R), such as stretching and/or walking.

A Sample Week of Exercise

Sunday: A relaxing activity, such as walking in nature or in a park; stretching (R).

Monday: Five minutes of stretching or low-impact aerobics (R), followed by a brisk walk, jog, or bicycle ride of at least twenty minutes (E) or some competitive game, such as tennis, racquetball, basketball (E). Followed by stretching (R).

Tuesday: Five minutes of stretching or low-impact aerobics (R), followed by a brisk walk, jog, or bicycle ride of at least twenty minutes (E) or some competitive game (E). Followed by stretching (R).

Wednesday: Five minutes of stretching or low-impact aerobics (R), followed by a brisk walk, jog, or bicycle ride of at least twenty minutes (E) or a competitive game (E). Stretching cooldown (R).

Thursday: Five minutes of stretching or low-impact aerobics (R), followed by a brisk walk, jog, or bicycle ride of at least twenty minutes (E) or some competitive game (E). Followed by stretching (R).

Friday: Optional exercise day. You can choose to do twenty minutes of stretching or some other R activity or combine an E and an R as described for Monday through Thursday.

Saturday: Twenty minutes of stretching, low-impact aerobics, strolling, fishing, canoeing, or some other relaxing activity (R).

Considerations for Your Exercise Plan

Remember that this part of your program is designed to bring about changes gradually. It will be most effective if you are consistent and follow it daily.

Strenuous exercise three to four times a week can cause an increase in baseline serotonin after thirty to forty-five days. This would be optimal for you. However, if you aren't able to do strenuous exercise that frequently, then you are better off following Program 1. If you feel stress or anxiety with daily cardiovascular exercise, try alternating your strenuous activity with stretching activities. You may also want to evaluate your competitiveness. If you find yourself being competitive, try to do alternative exercise programs that provide "inner challenges" instead of outer competition. Competitiveness can create stress if it results in your feeling like a failure. Occasional competitive activities, such as tennis or golf, may be fine if your self-esteem isn't at risk. Or if you enjoy competitive activities, play the "inner game." Set up personal standards to compete against, like walking a bit farther today than you did yesterday. Make those standards achievable and fun and you will enhance your self-esteem, thereby promoting an increase in serotonin.

Suggested Activities for Times of Stress, Anxiety, or Depression

Your brain chemistry is affected when you are under pressure or a great deal of stress. This may cause you to feel "out of balance," anxious, or depressed. Often depressed or down feelings are felt the day after a stressful event. Specific activities can be used to help balance your brain chemistry and thus help you feel and perform better.

When under stress, use an R activity followed by an E activity to help boost serotonin and "burn up" the excessive norepinephrine and dopamine caused by the stress.

If you follow this exercise program consistently, you should begin to notice an improvement in your ability to focus, your energy levels, and mood swings. Your anxiety or stress levels should also improve.

Tips for the Traveler

Often the person who must travel finds it difficult to maintain a consistent exercise program. The following are some tips you may want to consider to maintain consistency and peak performance.

1. Use the stairs instead of elevators.
2. A stroll or slow walk can serve as an ideal R type of activity for you.
3. Stay in hotels with pools and exercise facilities.
4. Schedule times to exercise; you'll feel better the next day.
5. Go for a walk in the morning and evening if possible. If the weather is bad or the area is unsafe, walk up and down the stairs a few times.
6. Stay in hotels within walking distance of your meetings, if at all possible. If the materials or accessories needed for your meeting are too heavy to carry, try to transport them in travel bags on wheels.

If you use a few of these simple suggestions, you won't have to "go somewhere else" to exercise unless you choose to do so.

Activities for the Satiation-Depressed Person

SEROTONIN-BOOSTING ACTIVITIES

1. Feel your feelings.
   - Write in a journal daily. Use the Pennebaker method.

- See a counselor or therapist.
- When you get into your car, check your feelings before you put the key in the ignition. Take a deep breath and relax. No matter what you feel, give yourself permission to have these emotions, passions, and desires. Confess your feelings to yourself and respond with acceptance and love.

2. Spend time in nature.
   - Start a hobby that involves the outdoors, such as hiking, camping, boating, canoeing, or fishing.
   - Walk in nature.
   - Garden.

3. Listen to serotonin-boosting music daily.
   - See Chapter Seven for suggestions.
   - Whenever you drive, turn on the radio or listen to serotonin-boosting tapes or CDs.

4. Adopt a spiritual or religious practice and adhere to it daily.
   - Meditate.
   - Pray throughout the day.
   - Attend some religious service or spiritual study group.

5. Know your trigger situations and defuse them by following the guidelines offered in Chapter Six.

If you are a Satiation-depressed person, the best way to start this program is by reexamining your life using the brain-chemistry model and then incorporating serotonin-boosting activities immediately. Do not pressure yourself to change. Rather, adopt the dietary program and do the serotonin-boosting activities every day, allowing these tools to change your brain chemistry and your mood. Consistency is important, but don't berate yourself when you deviate from the program. Get back on track as quickly as you can, and stay on the program for as long as you can. The more consistent you are in following this program, the quicker your baseline will change, and the sooner you will escape depression.

Chapter 9

A Program for Healing
Arousal Depression

General Treatment Approach

As we described in Chapter Five, if you are suffering from Arousal depression, you have low levels of serotonin and excessively high levels of norepinephrine and dopamine. Therefore, our strategy should be to raise your serotonin and gently lower your norepinephrine and dopamine. We can accomplish this by following these four general guidelines:

1. Adopt the brain-chemistry model for the Arousal-depressed personality, designed to balance your brain chemistry and help you overcome your depression.

2. Feel the feelings that exist below your anxiety. Do this gradually and in a way that you know to be safe. I recommend using a journal and writing daily, especially using the Pennebaker method.

3. Open up to a new way of living. One of the most effective and transformative insights we can have is the realization that we may have a blind spot about the solution to our problem. This means that the solution may exist, but we can't see it with our current set of attitudes and beliefs. We begin to change when we gently open up to new possibilities and new ways of being. The program described in this chapter can allow many new insights about yourself to bob up from below the surface. If practiced consistently, it can change your brain chemistry and your mood. The old beliefs that are currently holding you back will start to melt away so that you can see that you have more choices.

4. Understand that you have many needs that are currently going unmet. These contribute to your feelings of anxiety, depression, and lack of satisfaction with life. You can change this situation by following the program described here.

A Diet for the Arousal-Depressed Person

Before you start any diet program designed to help you relieve your anxiety and underlying depression, you need to recognize that as an Arousal personality type there are certain foods that have a particularly strong impact on your emotional health.

1. *Protein-rich foods.* Protein increases blood levels of tyrosine, which in turn promotes the production of norepinephrine and dopamine. The higher the protein content of your diet, the more anxiety, stress, and nervous tension you're going to experience. The more stress and anxiety you feel, the less you will be able to relax and deal with your underlying condition.

My Recommendation: In order to feel more calm, safe, and under control, you should gradually but significantly reduce protein-rich foods in your diet. Follow the guidelines provided here, and your protein intake will automatically fall to safer and more healthful levels.

2. *Caffeine.* One of the ways you are likely to maintain a state of high anxiety is through the use of caffeinated beverages and foods,

including coffee, tea, cola drinks, and chocolate. These foods keep your stress level up, and this distracts you from feeling your underlying condition.

My Recommendation: Significantly reduce or eliminate coffee and soft drinks. Various coffee substitutes, such as Caffix and Pero, can be drunk at night to provide a coffeelike flavor without the caffeine that will disturb your sleep.

3. *Refined carbohydrates,* such as white-flour products, sugar, and/or alcohol. In all likelihood, you are balancing your anxiety in a number of ways, especially with the use of refined carbohydrates.

My Recommendation: Significantly reduce or eliminate all refined-flour products, all refined white sugar, and all alcohol. Substitute whole-grain flour products for white-flour foods; use more natural sugars, such as fruit juices, barley malt, rice syrup, and maple syrup, instead of refined sugar; and drink nonalcoholic beer or wine, sparkling water, water, or fruit juice instead of alcohol.

These three aspects of your diet are pivotal to changing your emotional condition and restoring your health. You can make the changes in these three factors that you feel comfortable with, but the more you adhere to these recommendations, the more profound the effects will be on your inner state.

General Dietary Guidelines

The goal of this program is to increase serotonin and gently decrease norepinephrine and dopamine. The following general recommendations will accomplish this.

1. Reduce or eliminate all forms of red meat and eggs from your diet. Because you show a less than optimal level of serotonin, this suggestion is important, especially if you feel any signs or symptoms of low energy or depression.
2. Rely on fish, chicken, beans, and tofu for your protein needs.

3. Reduce your intake of animal foods to four times a week. After two to three weeks, reduce animal foods again to three times a week. If anxiety exists, reduce animal food intake to once or twice a week.

4. Include a whole-grain food or dish at every meal. This will boost your serotonin levels significantly.

5. Snack on whole grains and foods made of whole-grain flour, such as rice cakes, whole-grain cookies, popcorn, whole-grain pastries, and raisin bread.

6. Eliminate or significantly reduce all caffeinated beverages and foods, such as chocolate, coffee, and some teas.

A Daily Eating Plan

Whole grains. Twice a day. These are essential to your diet to increase serotonin. These include brown rice, barley, oats, millet, and others. Boil or pressure-cook them.

Whole-grain flour products. Daily. These include pastas, whole-wheat bread, rye bread, and whole-grain muffins, desserts, and snacks.

Puffed grains and cereals. When desired. These include Wheaties, Cheerios, Raisin Bran, and many others. If you would like to avoid dairy products, use soy milk or apple juice as a substitute for milk.

Green, leafy, and/or yellow vegetables. Once or twice daily. These include collard greens, kale, mustard greens, broccoli, and others.

Root vegetables. Two or three times a week. These include onion, celery, turnips, rutabagas, and others.

Fresh fruit. Daily. Dried fruits—whenever desired.

Fish. Two or three times a week. The list includes cod, scrod, flounder, halibut, salmon, and others. (All are low in fat; salmon contains omega polyunsaturated fats, which lower blood cholesterol.)

Chicken. Once a week. Remove the skin before eating.

Menu Suggestions

BREAKFAST

The following breakfast suggestions boost serotonin levels.

- Oatmeal with raisins or other fruit, or with honey or rice syrup
- Oatmeal mixed with bulgur wheat, rice, Wheatena, or other grains
- Leftover brown rice: the dinner rice can be reheated with more water to make it wetter and looser for the morning meal.
- Toast with jams (preferably those with no sugar added)
- Whole-grain muffin
- English muffin
- Hash browns
- Cereals, preferably with no added sugar: puffed rice and other puffed whole grains, Wheaties, Cheerios, Raisin Bran, and many others. If you would like to avoid dairy products, use apple juice as a substitute for milk.
- Fruit juice

The following breakfast foods will boost dopamine and norepinephrine levels, which can exacerbate the anxiety and depression of the Arousal personality. Therefore, the following breakfast foods should be minimized until the anxiety is reduced and depression is alleviated.

- Eggs
- Bacon, sausage, or other red meats
- Any type of fish or fish soup
- Smoked salmon (lox)

- Coffee
- Tea

LUNCH

The following lunch suggestions will boost serotonin levels.

- A whole grain: brown rice, millet, barley, and corn are among those listed in Chapter Seven.
- A green vegetable: collard greens, kale, mustard greens, turnip greens, and broccoli are among the best.
- A root or squash or other vegetable: this can include carrots, daikon radish, or some other vegetable listed in Chapter Seven.
- A piece of fresh fruit, preferably in season
- Leftover grain from dinner
- Sandwiches composed of whole-grain bread, leafy green vegetables (such as collard greens or kale), salad, mustard, balsamic vinegar, olive oil
- Pasta
- Hash brown potatoes
- Greens and mixed vegetable salad
- Lightly steamed or sautéed vegetables
- Vegetable soup, such as minestrone
- Whole-grain burgers, with a variety of toppings, on whole-grain bread or bun: available in stores, they need only be thawed and heated in the morning before work or at lunch.
- Wide variety of whole-grain chapati sandwiches, consisting of brown rice and vegetables wrapped in chapati: widely available in natural foods stores

The following lunch suggestions will boost dopamine and norepinephrine levels and may heighten the anxiety of the Arousal-depressed person. These foods should be minimized, at least until your anxiety is reduced significantly and your depression is alleviated.

- All forms of red meat, including luncheon meats
- Fish (allowed twice a week on the Arousal diet)
- Tuna salad sandwich
- Chicken, such as chicken or turkey salad sandwich (Chicken is allowed once a week on the Arousal diet.)

DINNER
The following dinner suggestions will boost serotonin levels.

- A whole grain, such as brown rice, wild rice, barley, millet (pressure-cooked or boiled), tabbouleh, others; with any number of condiments: many grains can be purchased pre-packaged and ready to be heated and served.
- Vegetable or grain soup
- Pasta: any one of a wide variety of noodles with marinara sauce or some other vegetable topping of your choice
- Steamed or sautéed leafy green vegetable
- Baked squash
- Baked potato
- Beans: bean burritos, bean tacos
- A root vegetable or vegetable medley that includes carrots, mushrooms, broccoli, and/or others
- Salad with a variety of leafy greens, celery, carrot, cucumber

The following dinner foods will boost dopamine and norepinephrine and therefore should be eaten in small amounts or less frequently through the course of the week, at least until your anxiety and depression are alleviated.

- All forms of red meat
- Chicken, turkey (allowed once a week on the Arousal diet)
- Fish (allowed twice a week on the Arousal diet)

Some General Thoughts About the Dietary Plan

In order to make the suggested dietary adjustments as easy and as comfortable as possible, I recommend that you gradually decrease foods that are rich in protein and refined carbohydrates, which may be contributing significantly to your current brain-chemistry imbalance. As you decrease the amount of red meat, eggs, and other high-fat, high-protein foods that you eat, increase vegetable foods, such as whole grains, fresh vegetables, beans, and fruit. These foods will balance your neurotransmitters and restore harmony to your inner state.

WHERE WILL I GET MY PROTEIN?

Many people worry whether they will get adequate protein if they begin to decrease the animal foods in their diet and increase whole grains, fresh vegetables, and beans. In fact, nutrition scientists point out that a completely vegetarian diet contains all the protein an adult needs to maintain optimal health.

Protein is used by the body for the creation of hormones, cell replacement and repair, and the production of body hair. In order to meet and exceed all of the body's requirements for protein, an adult must eat approximately twenty grams of protein a day, which amounts to about two-thirds of an ounce. You can get that much protein and more per day just by eating your fill of potatoes. I'm not suggesting that you eat only potatoes; the point is that as long as you eat a diet based largely on whole foods—such as whole, unrefined grains and vegetables, beans, and fruit—you cannot become deficient in protein, even if the diet is composed entirely of vegetables. All whole, unrefined vegetable foods contain complete protein. In fact, no nutritionist can create a diet made up of whole vegetable foods that is inadequate in protein, even for a child.

On the other hand, you do not need to become a vegetarian. Fish and poultry are rich sources of protein, though they should be used in limited quantities.

You can also adjust your protein intake to suit your own needs. Keep in mind, however, that most Americans today eat far too much protein to maintain their physical and mental health. Science has demonstrated that excess protein is linked to osteoporosis, kidney disorders, and several types of cancer. The National Academy of Sciences, the office of the U.S. surgeon general, and other prestigious scientific groups have encouraged Americans to reduce their intake of protein-rich foods and especially reduce the consumption of animal protein. The reason is simple: many of the animal sources of protein are high-fat foods, especially red meats, eggs, and many dairy products. The only exceptions to this are fish and the white meat of poultry. All animal foods have cholesterol, as well.

By eating large amounts of fat and protein, you increase your risk of a whole host of degenerative diseases, including heart disease, cancer, adult-onset diabetes, and other serious disorders. It may also contribute to your anxiety.

OTHER IMPORTANT CONSIDERATIONS

1. If a physician has suggested an alternative diet due to a medical condition or for any other reason, please follow that advice.

2. If you have food allergies, use alternative foods.

3. High-sodium foods may be inappropriate if you have high blood pressure or certain other medical conditions.

4. The goal of this diet is not to reduce your weight but to provide a balanced diet for your brain.

5. The body needs carbohydrates to function. Complex carbohydrates (such as whole grains, rice, potatoes, and pasta) are the most effective foods for increasing serotonin and maintaining balanced moods.

6. Eat at least three meals a day of the approved foods.

7. Avoid all alcohol and nonprescribed medications or drugs.

8. Trim all visible fat from poultry and fish.

9. Replace saturated fats with polyunsaturated fats and decrease the amount of fats consumed. To cut back on saturated fats, you can cut back on animal fats and trim excess fat from meat. It can also help to use cooking oils that are lower in saturated fats, such as canola or safflower oil. Remember that although margarine has lower saturated fat than butter, it is still a rather high-fat food.

10. Minimize your consumption of high-cholesterol foods.

11. Avoid or minimize your consumption of processed or refined sugars.

12. Minimize the use of salt and foods high in salt content.

13. Choose fresh foods over processed foods.

14. Avoid frying or immersing foods in oil; instead, broil, steam, or bake foods as much as possible.

15. Please consult your physician if you have any questions or suffer from other medical problems.

Your Daily Activity Plan

A Cautionary Note Before You Begin

Before you begin any exercise or activity program, you should consult your physician to determine if you have any physical limitations or preexisting conditions that could become worse with exercise. If after you begin your activity plan, your symptoms worsen or you feel more depressed or anxious, please discontinue the activity and consult your physician.

Research has shown that certain types of exercise and activities can have both immediate and long-term effects on brain chemistry and overall health. The program suggested here can enhance your brain chemistry when followed consistently. These suggestions are based on what I have found to be a generally safe and effective exercise program for an Arousal-depressed person. But you may need to modify the program somewhat to meet your individual needs, scheduling demands, and lifestyle. When making modifications, use the guidelines outlined in Chapters Three and Seven. In general, your exercise program should increase serotonin and reduce norepinephrine and dopamine.

General Guidelines for Your Exercise Program

There are two categories of exercise and activities that affect brain chemistry. The first type, called relaxing (designated with an "R"), boosts serotonin levels, while the second, called exciting (designated with an "E"), increases norepinephrine and dopamine if performed three times a week for six to eight weeks. Relaxing activities do not significantly increase your heart rate, while exciting activities tend to be aerobic or physically demanding. "E" activities performed occasionally will "burn up" dopamine and norepinephrine.

EXAMPLES OF "R" ACTIVITIES

Walking slow on a flat surface (strolling)

Biking on a flat surface

Camping

Canoeing

Stretching exercises

Fishing

Woodworking

See Chapter Seven for more "R," or serotonin-boosting, activities.

EXAMPLES OF "E" ACTIVITIES

Running

Mountain climbing

Hunting

Weight lifting

Swimming

Hiking

Aerobics

Racquet sports

Mountain biking

Competitive sports

See Chapter Seven for more "E," or norepinephrine-boosting, activities.

As you read these lists, pick out the ones you enjoy most, and consider how you can incorporate them into your schedule and lifestyle. Choose the ones you will be willing to do on a consistent basis. Next consider your present exercise schedule. How often are you doing an "R" activity? How often are you doing an "E" activity?

Exercise Program

The goal of this exercise program is to increase brain levels of serotonin and decrease dopamine and norepinephrine.

DAILY SCHEDULE

Sun.	Mon.	Tue.	Wed.	Thur.	Fri.	Sat.
R	E/R	R	E/R	R	E/R	R

Limit "E" activities to three times a week, and do not perform them two days in a row.

Exercise Program for People Not Exercising Now

Sun.	Mon.	Tue.	Wed.	Thur.	Fri.	Sat.
R	E/R	R	R	R	E/R	R

Perform a five-minute warm-up, such as stretching and walking, before doing an E exercise. Do twenty minutes of E or R exercises, and then another five minutes of cooldown activities, such as stretching and/or walking.

A Sample Week of Exercise

Sunday: A relaxing activity, such as walking in nature or in a park; stretching (R).

Monday: Twenty minutes of stretching warm-up (R). A brisk walk, jog, or bicycle ride of at least twenty minutes (E) or some competitive game, such as tennis, racquetball, basketball (E). Followed by stretching (R).

Tuesday: Stretching (R) or strolling (R) for at least twenty minutes.

Wednesday: Five minutes of stretching warm-up (R). A brisk walk, jog, or bicycle ride of at least twenty minutes (E) or a competitive game (E). Stretching cooldown (R).

Thursday: Stretching (R) or strolling (R) for at least twenty minutes.

Friday: Five minutes of stretching or low-impact aerobics (R). A brisk walk, jog, or bicycle ride of at least twenty minutes (E) or a competitive sport (E). Stretching as a cooldown (R).

Saturday: Stretching, low-impact aerobics, strolling, fishing, canoeing, or some other relaxing activity (R).

If you enjoy exercise and are already performing exciting or arousing exercise regularly, you can use the following schedule as your exercise routine.

SCHEDULE

Sun.	Mon.	Tue.	Wed.	Thur.	Fri.	Sat.
	E	E	E	E	E	

When you do "E" activities at least four times a week you increase serotonin, dopamine, and norepinephrine levels. However, for the vast majority of people the increase in serotonin is far greater than the increase in dopamine and norepinephrine. If you find that you feel anxious, cut down to two or three "E" activities a week. By exercising strenuously at least five days a week, you will elevate your serotonin levels. This elevation will counteract the effects of high dopamine.

Considerations for Your Exercise Plan

Remember that this part of your program is designed to bring about changes gradually. It will be most effective if you are consistent and follow it daily.

1. Strenuous exercise performed at least three to four times weekly can cause an increase in baseline serotonin after thirty to forty-five days. This would be optimal for you. However, if you aren't able to do strenuous exercise every day, then you can use daily stretching exercises. If you feel stress or anxiety with daily cardiovascular exercise, try alternating your strenuous activity with stretching activities. You may also want to evaluate your competitiveness. If you find yourself being competitive, try to do alternative exercise programs that provide "inner challenges" instead of outer competition. Competitiveness can create stress if it results in your feeling like a failure. Occasional competitive activities, such as tennis or golf, may be fine if your self-esteem isn't at risk. Or if you enjoy competitive activities, play the "inner game." Set up personal standards to compete against, like walking a bit

farther today than you did yesterday. Make those standards achievable and fun and you will enhance your self-esteem, thereby promoting an increase in serotonin.

2. If you aren't exercising at all, your serotonin levels are likely to remain low and your norepinephrine and dopamine will stay high, which means that you will probably be anxious and depressed. Try to get some exercise daily.

Suggested Activities for Times of Stress, Anxiety, or Depression

Your brain chemistry is affected when you are under pressure or a great deal of stress. This may cause you to feel "out of balance," anxious, or depressed. Often depressed or down feelings are felt the day after a stressful event. Specific activities can be used to help balance your brain chemistry and thus help you feel and perform better.

When under stress, use an E activity to help decrease elevated levels of dopamine. Perform this activity for at least twenty minutes, making sure you warm up beforehand and cool down afterward. This additional "E" exercise will tend to "burn up" unwanted norepinephrine and dopamine caused by stress.

If you follow this exercise program consistently, you should begin to notice an improvement in your ability to focus, your energy levels, and mood swings. Your anxiety or stress levels should also improve.

Tips for the Traveler

Often the person who must travel finds it difficult to maintain a consistent exercise program. The following are some tips you may want to consider to maintain consistency and peak performance.

1. Use the stairs instead of elevators.

2. A stroll or slow walk can serve as an ideal R type of activity for you.

3. Stay in hotels with pools and exercise facilities.

4. Schedule times to exercise; you'll feel better the next day.

5. Go for a walk in the morning and evening if possible. If the weather is bad or the area is unsafe, walk up and down the stairs a few times.

6. Stay in hotels within walking distance of your meetings, if at all possible. If the materials or accessories needed for your meeting are too heavy to carry, try to transport them in travel bags on wheels.

If you use a few of these simple suggestions, you won't have to "go somewhere else" to exercise unless you choose to do so.

Activities for the Arousal-Depressed Person

SEROTONIN-BOOSTING ACTIVITIES
THAT WILL ALSO LOWER NOREPINEPHRINE

1. Feel your feelings.
   - Write in a journal daily. Use the Pennebaker method.
   - See a counselor or therapist.
   - When you get into your car, check your feelings before you put the key in the ignition. Take a deep breath and relax. No matter what you feel, give yourself permission to have these emotions, passions, and desires. Confess your feelings to yourself and respond with acceptance and love.

2. Spend time in nature.
   - Start a hobby that involves the outdoors, such as hiking, camping, boating, canoeing, or fishing.
   - Walk in nature.
   - Garden.

3. Listen to serotonin-boosting music daily.
   - See Chapter Seven for suggestions.

- Whenever you drive, turn on the radio or listen to serotonin-boosting tapes or CDs.

4. Adopt a spiritual or religious practice and adhere to it daily.

   - Meditate.

   - Pray throughout the day.

   - Attend some religious service or spiritual study group.

5. Know your trigger situations and defuse them by following the guidelines offered in Chapter Six.

If you are an Arousal-depressed person, the best way to start this program is by examining your life using the brain-chemistry model and then incorporating serotonin-boosting and dopamine-decreasing activities immediately. Be especially careful of competitiveness. Whenever you feel pressure to win, do serotonin-boosting and dopamine-depleting activities. Do not pressure yourself to change. Instead, adopt the dietary program and do the serotonin-enhancing and dopamine-suppressing activities every day. Consistency is important, but don't berate yourself when you deviate from the program. Get back on track as quickly as you can, and stay on the program for as long as you can. The more consistent you are in following this program, the more quickly your baseline will change and the sooner you will escape depression and anxiety.

Chapter 10

Restoring Balance
as a Practical Tool
for Healing

D epression challenges us to think about health and
illness in new ways. Using the brain-chemistry
model, we can see that depression is an imbal-
ance in our neurochemistry, nutrition, behavior, and outlook on life.
The sheer scope of the imbalance would seem daunting if it were
not for the fact that the brain-chemistry model also gives us practical
tools for successfully addressing and healing this imbalance.

To the hard scientist and medical doctor, "imbalance" may be an
off-putting term. It may conjure up images that are long on sympathy
and short on therapeutic value. But in fact, "balance" is an old term in
the healing arts. Its use goes back to Hippocrates, who established the
first scientific approach to medicine. For the "father of medicine,"
health involved the balancing of four aspects of the body that he called

"humors." Disease, on the other hand, arose from an imbalance among these elements in the body and, indeed, in the person's life.

Interestingly, Hippocrates saw that illness offers an opportunity to establish a new and higher degree of health, or what he called a new "blended maturity." Disease, he noted, is an organic and orderly process that when treated correctly can serve to eliminate what is old and useless—a process he called *katharsis*. At a certain point in the development of an illness, the physician is able to intervene on the patient's behalf; this is the moment Hippocrates referred to as a healing "crisis" (*krisis* in the Greek). At that moment, the physician's job is to arrange the internal and environmental elements in such a way that they assist the body, mind, and spirit in establishing a new balance—a "blended maturity" (*krasis* in the Greek).

The brain-chemistry model is a product of the most modern scientific knowledge. Indeed, much of what we know of brain chemistry has been discovered only in the past twenty years or so. Yet despite its cutting-edge nature, the model harks back to the roots of medicine, offering us a chance to utilize the old tool of balance in a modern and highly effective way. We are now challenged to balance neurotransmitters rather than "humors," with a special focus on the big three brain chemicals: serotonin, norepinephrine, and dopamine. And just as Hippocrates manipulated internal and environmental circumstances to restore balance, so must we. Indeed, as we learn more about brain chemistry and specifically about these three neurochemicals, we begin to understand how our daily behavior influences them and how useful balance can be as a guiding therapeutic tool.

But balance can only be restored with the individual's assistance and full participation, which is as it should be. After all, depression is as much a mental and spiritual crisis as it is a physical one. If we are to treat the condition effectively, we must enlist the person's body, mind, and spirit in the struggle to achieve balance. Practically speaking, this means that the person who suffers from depression must address areas of life that he or she has consciously or unconsciously avoided. And he or she must adopt new and more balanced behaviors and ways of looking at life.

As I have said throughout this book, the underlying cause of depression is an imbalance among neurochemicals. This imbalance is sustained or overcome by what we do each day, which includes the foods we eat, the activities we engage in, and the thoughts that we maintain consistently. All of our activities can be categorized along the Satiation-Arousal continuum. Depression arises when our daily behavior is consistently one-sided—either too much of the Satiation type or too much of the Arousal. Either imbalance can give rise to its own type of depression; though both are labeled depression, each is a very different condition.

All of us are driven by the need for safety, security, and consistency in life, and these are essential for mental health. Yet each of us is confronted with an underlying paradox: as we pursue safety and consistency, we are continually being compelled to grow beyond our current limits—in our relationships, our jobs, and even our belief systems. Indeed, science teaches us that growth, maturity, and adaptation are essential to our survival. If we tend to be Satiation types by nature, life seems to compel us to adopt a certain number of Arousal behaviors in order to remain healthy and fully alive. If we are Arousal types by nature, health demands that we incorporate a certain number of Satiation behaviors in our daily life. To remain fixed at one or the other extreme—either Satiation or Arousal—is to stagnate, decline, and eventually fall into depression. To grow beyond our current limits is to adapt, to be refreshed, to achieve a new "blended maturity."

As I stressed in Chapter One, the current means of treatment, including drugs and psychotherapy, are often essential in dealing with depression, especially when the illness places a person's life in danger. In fact, these therapies can also be seen as having their place along the Satiation-Arousal continuum. But in order to make a true recovery, scientists, physicians, and the depressed patient must embrace a larger understanding of the illness, of health, and of life itself.

Life is pushing each of us to grow, adapt, and achieve balance. Depression occurs when we resist these demands. Yet this condition can be overcome by restoring balance in our thinking, nutrition, and daily activities. Hippocrates saw that within any disorder lie the seeds for renewal. Depression is no different. No matter how dark our mood or circumstances may be, there is at the center of our lives a light that keeps us alive, that keeps telling us that today's limits are not tomorrow's, and that we have the power to change and thus find our way out of the darkness.

The brain-chemistry model, as I have described it, is a step toward that light—the light of balance and the restoration of health.

Robertson Institute Mood Optimization Survey^{sm}

Clinical Version

Ｉf you are interested in receiving a more detailed evalu-
ation and plan to optimize your moods, we offer you
the Robertson Mood Optimization Program. This
program is a comprehensive report of thirty-five to forty pages offering
you information about your brain chemistry and specific diet, exercise,
spiritual, and behavior plans for your recovery. This program is tailored
specifically to you. For example, we use at least 1,260 different dietary
plans to tailor your recovery program. The program requires you to
complete the following survey and return it to our offices.

The survey attached to this book has a special marking that will
give you $20.00 off the list price as a token of appreciation for purchas-
ing the book. Please include $39.95 (regular price $59.95; Michigan
residents add 6 percent sales tax), plus $4.55 for shipping and handling.

Instructions for Completing the Survey

1. Please complete all information on the top of the answer sheet,
   including your name, address, phone number, and method of
   payment.

2. Completely fill in the appropriate circle for each question.

3. Take your time and read all the questions thoroughly.

4. Your answers should reflect your feelings over the past year, rather than over the last few days or weeks, unless otherwise stated.

5. Please answer every question.

6. If you are not sure of an answer, choose the closest "true" or "false" answer.

7. If a question doesn't pertain to you or you can't determine if it is true or false, answer it "false."

8. Questions relating to alcohol or drug usage are not for the purpose of determining abuse but rather for measuring the effects these substances have on the brain.

9. There are no wrong answers, good answers, or bad answers, just honest answers. Please be honest.

After completing the survey, please send your answer sheet along with payment to Robertson Institute, Ltd., Testing Division, 3555 Pierce St., Saginaw, MI 48604. Australian residents should send the answer sheet and payment to Robertson Institute, Ltd., P.O. Box 615, North Sydney, NSW 2059.

Robertson Institute Mood Optimization Survey[sm]

1. I prefer being alone to being with others.

2. I am a "down" person or somewhat depressed.

3. One or more of my brothers, sisters, parents, or grandparents now has, or has had, arthritis or stiffness in their joints. (If you are adopted, answer this question "false.")

4. I often feel angry.

5. I spend money or buy things when I am "down," angry, or nervous.

6. I participate in group activities that have consistent guidelines and provide emotional fulfillment.

7. I watch television or read more than fifteen hours a week.

8. I find it hard to have a comfortable relationship with other people.

9. My friends or family have confronted me about spending too much time working or being busy.

10. I now have difficulty remembering things I used to be able to remember easily.

11. I become angry when I am depressed or anxious.

12. It bothers me when someone does something better than I do.

13. I watch television, movies, or videos more than four hours a day at least four days a week.

14. I feel that many people dislike me.

15. One or more of my brothers, sisters, parents, or grandparents now has, or has had, high blood pressure. (If you are adopted, answer this question "false.")

16. One or more of my brothers, sisters, parents, or grandparents now has, or has had, Alzheimer's disease or early senility. (If you are adopted, answer this question "false.")

17. I have recently experienced at least one of the four following conditions: chest pains, shortness of breath, blue fingernails, or dizziness when I stand up.

18. I have trouble being with people because I feel insecure.

19. I find myself overreacting to situations when I get stressed or depressed.

20. One or more of my children may have a problem with alcoholism, gambling, drug addiction, or overeating. (If you have no children, answer this question "false.")

21. I continue to eat even after I am full.

22. I have lost more than ten pounds in thirty days without dieting.

23. People have told me that I work too much or that I am overinvolved in things.

24. I prefer to spend time with a small group of people rather than a large group of people.

25. I am more comfortable knowing lots of people rather than having a few close friends.

26. I should "slow down" because I feel there is no need to push myself so fast or to do the exciting things I do.

27. During this past year, I have felt more muscle weakness than before.

28. During this past year, I have experienced changes in my desire or need for exciting activities.

29. I watch exciting movies or videos or play computer games more than fifteen hours a week.

30. I experience ringing in my ears.

31. To help me relax, I have used medication, alcohol, or some other substance.

32. I experience a significant change in my mood at least three times a week.

33. When I am frustrated, angry, depressed, or stressed, I eat even though I am not hungry.

34. When I am with people in a social setting, I am usually one of the last to leave.

35. I enjoy strenuous exercise two to four times a week.

36. I dislike exercise.

37. When I am stressed or anxious, I like to do exciting things to help me calm down.

38. One to three of my brothers, sisters, parents, or grandparents has, or has had, a problem with alcoholism, gambling, drug addiction, or overeating. (If you are adopted, answer this question "false.")

39. I am fearful or insecure.

40. Even a small amount of anxiety makes me feel uncomfortable.

41. When I am depressed, I have trouble getting started on projects that need to be completed.

42. Four or more of my biological aunts, uncles, or cousins have, or have had, a problem with alcoholism, gambling, drug addiction, or overeating. (If you are adopted, answer this question "false.")

43. I like behaviors or activities that give me a "lift" or make me feel better.

44. I prefer highly competitive, goal-oriented activities over those that involve quiet self-reflection.

45. If I feel someone will question my ideas, I will try to avoid discussing them.

46. I like exercise that tones my muscles more than exercise that makes me sweat.

47. I watch television or videos, go to the movies, and/or listen to music or tapes more than fifteen hours per week.

48. People have told me that I clean or organize my home, office, or possessions too much.

49. I struggle with procrastination.

50. I have been hospitalized or have had medication prescribed for depression or "feeling down."

51. I often spend more than I earn in a month.

52. I often take part in activities that involve high risk, such as whitewater rafting, mountain climbing, or driving fast cars.

53. I like to socialize with large groups of people.

54. I find myself trying to control people and situations when I get nervous, depressed, or stressed.

55. I usually don't get anxious or nervous in social settings.

56. I am a loner.

57. I have gambled (including risky financial investments) despite financial difficulties.

58. I have trouble sleeping through the night, even if not interrupted, at least four times a week.

59. I can confront people easily when I feel they have done me wrong.

60. I watch television, read, or meditate less than five hours a week.

61. I accept criticism well.

62. I watch action-oriented or competitive sports programs at least fifteen hours a week.

63. I have been more than thirty pounds overweight.

64. I get depressed or feel down if I don't do my best.

65. I have seen things that were not real when I was not drinking alcohol or on medication.

66. I am more than fifty pounds overweight.

67. I like being with others more than being alone.

68. I like groups, including religious groups, that have clear standards, rules, or codes of behavior.

69. I experience pounding in my head, headaches, or sinus pain at least twice a week.

70. When I am depressed or feel down, I feel like I have to accomplish something to make myself feel better.

71. When I feel down, I may use drugs or alcohol to help me feel better.

72. I lose energy the longer I am with a large group of people.

73. I feel depressed or down when I am not accomplishing something.

74. I have recently begun to forget the names of people, places, and things.

75. I buy things that I don't need, even when I feel I can't afford them.

76. I have difficulty focusing my eyes, or I often see double.

77. I have a problem with controlling people or situations.

78. I like risky activities such as speeding, mountain climbing, hang gliding, and racing.

79. I use exciting activities to make me feel better when I am down.

80. I participate in risky activities in spite of having been injured while doing them in the past.

81. I fear people, places, or things.

82. I am more than thirty pounds but less than fifty pounds overweight.

83. When I disagree with someone, I usually remain silent.

84. I have a difficult time remaining friends with people who disagree with me.

85. I have trouble getting to sleep, even when I feel tired, at least four times a week.

86. I am stressed or nervous.

87. I am a very calm person.

88. When I feel stressed or nervous, I drink alcohol or use drugs to make myself feel better.

89. I experience diarrhea or nausea frequently.

90. I drink alcoholic beverages or use drugs or medication to give me energy when I feel down.

91. I have an irregular or rapid heart rate, or I sweat, without exercising.

92. I prefer to watch relaxing movies, videos, or television programs rather than action, horror, or violent movies, videos, or television programs.

93. I usually spend my free time alone.

94. I now have or have had seizures or convulsions.

95. I have recently felt a general tiredness.

96. I would like to have several sexual partners.

97. I crave sweets, carbohydrates, or other sugar-based products when I am nervous, stressed, depressed, or angry.

98. I have trouble expressing my true feelings to those I care about.

99. I drink alcoholic beverages or use drugs when I become depressed.

100. I usually will drink alcoholic beverages or use drugs when I am with people in a social setting, if they are available.

101. I have been hospitalized or have had medication prescribed for anxiety or nervousness.

102. One of my brothers, sisters, parents, or grandparents now has, or has had, cancer. (If you are adopted, answer this question "false.")

103. I prefer to do relaxing activities alone rather than with a large group of people.

104. I prefer mild exercise to strenuous exercise.

105. I feel the need to clean my room, apartment, or home when I am depressed, angry, or nervous.

106. I am unable to relax when my room, apartment, or home needs simple cleaning.

107. One or more of my brothers, sisters, parents, or grandparents now has, or has had, epilepsy or convulsions. (If you are adopted, answer this question "false.")

108. I usually don't do things as well as I want to.

109. When I make a small mistake, I experience mood swings.

110. I have gained more than ten pounds in thirty days.

111. I prefer exercise that makes my heart beat faster over mild exercise.

112. I find myself feeling uncomfortable when things don't go the way I want them to.

113. I am sad.

114. When I make a small mistake, it takes me a while to forget about it.

115. I feel that I am too busy or work too hard to be able to relax as much as I would like.

116. My violent behavior or temper has caused my relationships to suffer.

117. I crave sweets, carbohydrates, or sugar-based products when I am nervous or stressed.

118. I do quieting activities to relax myself.

119. When I am asked to participate in activities where there is a winner, I feel nervous.

120. I need the approval of others or I get depressed.

121. It takes a great deal of frustration or conflict to make me feel nervous or stressed.

122. I purchase lottery tickets or bet on sporting events.

123. I usually watch movies, videos, or television programs or play computer games that involve action or excitement.

124. I experience significant mood swings on a daily basis.

125. I feel excited or good about myself when I gamble.

126. I am an angry person.

127. I am now, or have been, overweight.

128. I am stressed.

129. I use sex to relieve my frustrations or stress.

130. I am now, or have been, underweight.

131. I get bored having sex with the same person after a while.

132. I get constipated frequently.

133. I have taken prescribed medication, drunk alcohol, or used drugs to make myself feel better.

134. I have trouble staying awake during the day.

135. I do not drink alcohol, use drugs, or take prescribed medication.

136. I drink alcoholic beverages or use drugs even when I am not in a social setting. (Answer this "false" if you don't use alcohol or drugs.)

137. Quiet activities relax me.

138. When I drink alcohol, it calms me down.

139. I watch noncompetitive programs or events at least fifteen hours a week.

140. I have trouble urinating, have pain when I urinate, or have frequent urination.

141. I often wake up earlier than I would like.

142. I am an optimistic person.

143. I enjoy activities that require a lot of energy and excitement.

144. One or more of my brothers, sisters, parents, or grandparents is, or has been, more than twenty pounds but less than fifty pounds overweight. (If you are adopted, answer this question "false.")

145. I often have nasal or sinus congestion.

146. I am a positive person.

147. I enjoy spending time with a small group of people talking and sharing my feelings.

148. I worry about my health because of the amount of stress I am feeling.

149. One or more of my brothers, sisters, parents, or grandparents now has, or has had, heart problems. (If you are adopted, answer this question "false.")

150. I get stressed or nervous rather easily.

151. When I make a mistake and am confronted, I try to avoid the issue or make up excuses.

152. One or more of my brothers, sisters, parents, or grandparents is, or has been, at least fifty pounds overweight. (If you are adopted, answer this question "false.")

153. I have become angry and felt out of control more than once.

154. I enjoy competitive activities.

155. I prefer having a few close relationships to knowing a lot of people.

156. I have been put on probation at my work or feel I wasn't promoted because of my personal actions.

157. I enjoy watching or participating in violent activities.

158. I crave sweets, carbohydrates, or sugar-based products when I am down or depressed.

159. People close to me complain about my procrastination.

160. I drink alcohol or use drugs that alter my mood at least four times a week.

161. I prefer activities in which I can be an active participant over activities in which I am a spectator.

162. I prefer activities in which I can be a spectator over activities in which I am an active participant.

163. I have had hallucinations or heard voices or sounds when I was not drinking alcohol or using drugs.

164. I watch television, movies, or videos more than fifteen hours a week.

165. Food, alcohol, or other substances, including prescription drugs, that decrease my nervousness or stress make me feel better.

166. People do not support me or believe in me.

167. I find it difficult to concentrate because of my stress levels.

168. I have recently had a loss of appetite.

169. One of my brothers, sisters, parents, or grandparents now has, or has had, diabetes. (If you are adopted, answer this question "false.")

170. I tend to spend less time with people who disagree with me.

171. I have tried to lose weight in the past and failed.

172. I like to bet on a game in order to add excitement.

173. I suffer from one or more of the following: compulsiveness, being overweight, being underweight, depression, anxiety, mood swings.

174. I have a history of one or more of the following: heart disease, high blood pressure, high cholesterol, diabetes, other major medical condition.

175. According to my doctor, my overall health is excellent or above average.

176. I am an active person under the age of forty-five years, with no history of heart disease in the family and no medical conditions.

177. I am a semiactive or active person between the ages of forty-six and sixty-five years of age with no medical conditions.

178. I am relatively inactive or have medical conditions that will interfere with my health.

179. I have medically prescribed restrictions in my diet.

180. I have medically prescribed restrictions on my exercise or activity.

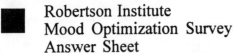

Robertson Institute
Mood Optimization Survey
Answer Sheet

44134

First Name: _____   Last Name: _____

Street Address: _____

City: _____   State: _____   Zip Code: _____

Country: _____   Phone #: _____   Fax #: _____

Method of Payment: _____   Credit Card Number: _____

Expiration Date: _____   Gender: _____   Age: _____

Completely fill in the appropriate circle for each question.

T F	T F	T F	T F	T F	T F
1 ○○	31 ○○	61 ○○	91 ○○	121 ○○	151 ○○
2 ○○	32 ○○	62 ○○	92 ○○	122 ○○	152 ○○
3 ○○	33 ○○	63 ○○	93 ○○	123 ○○	153 ○○
4 ○○	34 ○○	64 ○○	94 ○○	124 ○○	154 ○○
5 ○○	35 ○○	65 ○○	95 ○○	125 ○○	155 ○○
6 ○○	36 ○○	66 ○○	96 ○○	126 ○○	156 ○○
7 ○○	37 ○○	67 ○○	97 ○○	127 ○○	157 ○○
8 ○○	38 ○○	68 ○○	98 ○○	128 ○○	158 ○○
9 ○○	39 ○○	69 ○○	99 ○○	129 ○○	159 ○○
10 ○○	40 ○○	70 ○○	100 ○○	130 ○○	160 ○○
11 ○○	41 ○○	71 ○○	101 ○○	131 ○○	161 ○○
12 ○○	42 ○○	72 ○○	102 ○○	132 ○○	162 ○○
13 ○○	43 ○○	73 ○○	103 ○○	133 ○○	163 ○○
14 ○○	44 ○○	74 ○○	104 ○○	134 ○○	164 ○○
15 ○○	45 ○○	75 ○○	105 ○○	135 ○○	165 ○○
16 ○○	46 ○○	76 ○○	106 ○○	136 ○○	166 ○○
17 ○○	47 ○○	77 ○○	107 ○○	137 ○○	167 ○○
18 ○○	48 ○○	78 ○○	108 ○○	138 ○○	168 ○○
19 ○○	49 ○○	79 ○○	109 ○○	139 ○○	169 ○○
20 ○○	50 ○○	80 ○○	110 ○○	140 ○○	170 ○○
21 ○○	51 ○○	81 ○○	111 ○○	141 ○○	171 ○○
22 ○○	52 ○○	82 ○○	112 ○○	142 ○○	172 ○○
23 ○○	53 ○○	83 ○○	113 ○○	143 ○○	173 ○○
24 ○○	54 ○○	84 ○○	114 ○○	144 ○○	174 ○○
25 ○○	55 ○○	85 ○○	115 ○○	145 ○○	175 ○○
26 ○○	56 ○○	86 ○○	116 ○○	146 ○○	176 ○○
27 ○○	57 ○○	87 ○○	117 ○○	147 ○○	177 ○○
28 ○○	58 ○○	88 ○○	118 ○○	148 ○○	178 ○○
29 ○○	59 ○○	89 ○○	119 ○○	149 ○○	179 ○○
30 ○○	60 ○○	90 ○○	120 ○○	150 ○○	180 ○○

Signature _____